Endorsements for
Despite Your Circumstances

"With raw vulnerability, Candida brings us into her world of physical and psychological hardships. She shows us how she, with the help and strong faith in God, transcends her limitations and goes for the possibilities. *Despite Your Circumstances* shows us the power of the mind as it embraces an attitude of positivity and gratitude and shows us how we can build a rich life filled with meaning and joy beyond our challenging circumstances."
Harriet Cabelly, Social Worker & Life Coach at Rebuild Life Now

"Candida's book *Despite Your Circumstances* beautifully illustrates the human struggle to overcome circumstances beyond our control. The transformative power of God's love and radical acceptance leap off the pages."
Jason Kishpaugh, LPC-MHSP, Licensed Professional Mental Health Counselor

"I love how this book encourages us all to defeat the negative thoughts and change them to positive, God thoughts. This is a true lesson on how to transform your perspective on life circumstances."
Beth Stewart, founder of *Triumphant Living* radio ministry, CEO of Beth Stewart Ministries, and author of *Dreams NEVER Expire*

"This book will forever change your perspective by showing you how to shift your thinking to live a positive victorious life empowered by God. It will challenge you to rise above circumstances and remind you that as you think, so shall it be."
Terri Meredith, Terri Meredith Ministries

Despite Your Circumstances

Candida Sullivan

Copyright @ 2014 ShadeTree Publishing, LLC

Print ISBN: 978-1-937331-68-9

e-Book ISBN: 978-1-937331-69-6

Scripture quotations are taken from the King James Version, which is public domain in the United States.

All rights reserved. This book is protected by copyright. No part of this book may be reproduced or transmitted in any form or by any means, electronic or mechanical, including photocopying, recording, or by any information storage and retrieval system, without permission in writing from the publisher.

The purpose of this book is to educate and enlighten. This book is sold with the understanding that the publisher and author are not engaged in rendering counseling, albeit it professional or lay, to the reader or anyone else. The author shall have neither liability nor responsibility to any person or entity with respect to any loss or damage caused, or alleged to have been caused, directly or indirectly, by the information contain in this book.

Visit our Web site at www.ShadeTreePublishing.com.

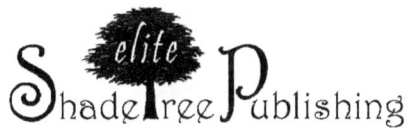

To my sister, Emily.

May you always jump in puddles and dance in the rain.

CONTENTS

Introduction	1
1 Determination and Motivation	5
2 Eye of Faith	13
3 Positive Versus Negative	21
4 Overcoming Stress	29
5 A Mile in My Shoes	37
6 God's Creativity	43
7 Making a Difference	49
8 Testing Times	57
9 Running Our Race	65
10 Our Stories	71
11 Fear	77
12 Great Expectations	85
13 Suffering with a Smile	93
14 Unconditional Happiness	99
15 Bad Days	103
16 My Big Change	107
Favorite Scriptures	113
About the Author	125
Other Books by Candida	126
About Amniotic Band Syndrome	131
Author's Acknowledgments	133

Candida Sullivan

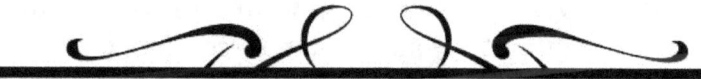

Introduction

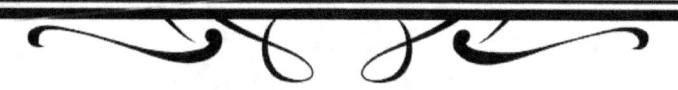

No one enjoys hardships. We may learn to appreciate their value, but at that moment, when the trial is ever-present and difficult to endure, we all wish for an easier way. If given options, we would all check the box that requires the least amount of suffering, pain, troubles, and trials. Most of us want a life of ease and glamour. No one elects health problems, financial burdens, grief, or any type of heartache as their way of life. Hardships often catch us unaware. They strike and leave us vulnerable and weak. In our weakened state, the seeds of self-doubt and pity emerge. They have no respect of persons and they try to destroy us all.

Any time the enemy can knock us down, he happily will. Then he will kick us and delight in our suffering. The louder we cry, the more control and power he has over us.

He capitalizes on our weaknesses and uses them against us. During the midst of our suffering, if hope diminishes, then we will feel defeated, alone, and frightened.

But just when it seems our heartaches and despair will swallow us whole, God intervenes, and His still, small voice whispers peace to our heart and courage to our soul. It is not His will that we be defeated. God wants us to walk in faith and trust Him. Regardless of His strength and power, God always gives us the freedom of choice. He allows us to decide if we want help or if we want to continue in our misery. It is ultimately our decision—comfort or distress; happiness or sadness.

Sometimes we forget we have a choice in life and tend to see only the bad in our lives. In our despair, we give up too easily and label things as being hopeless, when, in reality, our lives just need more effort. <u>Life is hard</u>! It will always be hard, and there is no enchanting formula to make it easier. *Or could there be?*

The difference between happiness and sadness is nothing more than perspective. The way we choose to look at life is exactly how it will be. We can walk around with our heads dropped, complaining about all that we've had to endure, or we can hold our heads up high and tell everyone we meet about our wonderful God, and how He helped us survive the storm.

We have all been smiled upon by God. He supplies our every need—in the good times and in the bad. The difference is that some people know when they are blessed, while others neglect to be thankful. Pessimistic people have their minds made up to be victims, and they refuse to allow anything or anyone to persuade them otherwise. At some point we all play the self-pity card and relish in the fact that others do pity us. We all dwell on events from the past, and we allow the bad to overpower the good, as well as dictate our future. If we look, there will always be a million excuses for not being happy, and most often times, we fight against happiness with every effort.

The devil will give us all a long list of reasons to not serve God. He has an abundance of reasons to justify bad behavior. The enemy can always make things seem hopeless. I know this because I believed the bad, negative thoughts of self-destruction for most of my life. I often relented as my mind became plagued with doubts and fears, and even surrendered as the enemy tried to destroy me with negative, doubtful thoughts. Then one day, God showed me that I'm capable of so much more than I even realized. I can reach whatever plateau in life I strive for. It all comes down to deciding how badly I want it, and then figuring out whether I'm willing to suffer, if that's what it takes to do the task.

This book is my story about overcoming and conquering my pessimistic self. It tackles some of my toughest, everyday challenges and demonstrates how God can transform us into stronger vessels for Him. The storms of our lives may not end, but God can certainly show us how to conquer them all. Serving God is the secret to happiness. Despite my circumstances, God can use me for His purposes. When I look to God and keep my eyes on Him, all I can see is the good.

Each chapter in this book ends with questions for us to think about and ponder, and when we are ready—to answer. Everyone can strive to be better. We all have areas in our life that need work, and this book is designed to be a tool to help us do that. I'm amazed at how much my life has been transformed in the last few years. I love these positive, happy changes and want to increase my wisdom, knowledge, and understanding even more.

I desire to fulfill my purpose while here on earth. I often reflect on my life and hope that God is pleased with me. I never want Him to be grieved that He allowed me to live on this planet. In order to reach my full potential and be fruitful for Him, I have to be willing to advance in my journey.

Not every moment of our travels is pleasant. We all reach valleys that test our strength and determination, and make us want to give up. It is during these times that we need to remember our purpose and keep progressing for the greater good of our lives.

I hope this book helps you in some way as it has helped me. I am happier, more productive, and have a better outlook on life than ever before, due to the lessons and skills documented in these pages. Through my Lord, I am an overcomer. May God bless you and your journey!

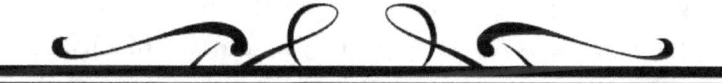

1
Determination and Motivation

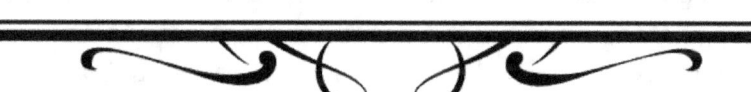

I can do all things through Christ which strengtheneth me.

                              Philippians 4:13

One day my life was a semblance of normal, and the next, my whole world shifted and twirled out of control. Without warning or a chance to prepare, bad news sucked me into a whirlwind of negativity and sorrow. It whittled away at my self-worth and even had me questioning my desire to live. No one wants to live in constant, debilitating pain.

The doctor painted a picture of hopelessness, complete with despair and defeat. According to my unique prognosis, I would never recover any balance of good health. My life had been cursed and plagued with one bad thing after another.

It all started with an attack of amniotic bands in my mother's womb. In all reality, these bands destroyed my chance at normalcy and caused the boomerang effect of health problems. Inflammation and arthritis felt as if it had entered every inch and joint of my body. Cysts formed and pressed on my nerves. The balance of my arms, caused by constant modifications, challenged me even more. Normal things, like taking a shower and driving, were extremely difficult— even on the good days. On top of all that, one day numbness attacked my legs and it became extremely hard for me to walk. It is one thing to be told these types of things might happen, but it is another thing completely when they actually occur.

Negative thoughts and fear of the unknown pushed me deeper into despair. I searched for hope on the Internet, only to be depressed even more. To read, in black and white, the fears of my heart erased what little hope I had left. At one point, it seemed my life was over.

Disabled. Handicapped. Defective. That's what doctor after doctor concurred. According to their knowledge of my condition, I would only get worse. Give up or keep trying to prove them wrong—these were my only options. In that moment of fear and heartache, I decided with my whole heart to fight back.

This was my life and I would not let anyone or anything take it from me! God had spared me from the bands in my mother's womb, and He has a plan for me. I wasn't finished yet. In all reality, we were just getting started—God and me.

Instead of signing up for my disability check, I joined the gym. The first time I tried to exercise, I cried the whole time. But instead of allowing the tears to stop or hinder me, I used them for my benefit. They fueled my determination and strengthened my spirit. The second workout was more of the same—tears and lots of pain. Regardless of the struggle, I didn't give up. Looking at myself in the mirror forced me to try harder. I dared my reflection to give up. Finally, I felt in control of the situation—with options and choices. I refused all pain medications and drugs. Vitamins and natural products that would heal my body seemed the better option. Then, of course, I decided to alter my diet for my particular conditions and health.

My new direction forced me to look at my life and health in different ways. I was no longer eating to satisfy my hunger and cure my cravings, but rather to fuel my body with the necessary energy to move toward wellness. My next trip to the grocery store was accompanied by panic and tears. Surrounded by food, I no longer knew what to purchase. I had to push aside all of my preconceived notions of what was healthy. For example, the wheat bread I thought was good for me actually contained a protein called gluten that was making me sick. As I scanned the aisles, forbidden foods overwhelmed me. Right there in the middle of the grocery store, I had to give myself a pep talk.

Yes, this is hard, but it's not impossible. You will get through this. It's only food! You still have the ability to eat, so stop whining and find the best quality food for your body. You've come too far to give up now!

One step, with determination and faith, was all I needed to move beyond the first initial shock. Instead of a sausage biscuit for breakfast, I had Greek yogurt and walnuts. Not only did the change in food make me feel better, but the knowledge that I was transforming myself into a better person from the inside out also gave me strength.

I learned to incorporate more fruits and vegetables into my diet and eat less saturated fat and sugar. Reading labels and deciding, with every bite or drink, if it was helpful or harmful to me forced me to make healthier choices. I'm not saying that I never eat anything bad anymore. Occasionally I do get off track, but still I always read labels and learn the contents of my food before I eat it. I do care what goes into my body, and I realize that everything—both the good and the bad—affect me.

I will never forget the day when I ripped my favorite jeans. I had ventured off of my healthy lifestyle and gained a few pounds. Of course I noticed the weight gain, but I told myself, over and over, that I didn't care. When I struggled to button my jeans and then tore a gaping hole in them, I burst into tears and realized that I did care—very much. Every single day, I have to do what is best for me.

I have a love-hate relationship with exercising. My body loves when I take the time to pamper and nurture it. Any effort, large or small, does incredible things for my health and makes my pain ease, causing my mood to brighten. Accomplishing goals makes me feel good about myself and advances me to places I never dreamed possible. When I overcome my own limitations, I feel alive and well.

Exercising is something I do for myself, every day. Well, except for the days when I talk myself into snoozing and think of many excuses to skip it. Those are the days when I drag. My mood teeters toward depression, and stress threatens to overtake me. Pain strikes with a vengeance and sends me back to bed. And then, while lying there in my misery, I start feeling sorry for myself.

Even though I know the problems and the solutions to them, still I find myself ignoring the things I need to do. Why? Because exercise is hard. It takes effort. Training takes strength, stamina, motivation, and dedication, all of which require that I dig deep and push myself. Reshaping my body as well as my mind is something I have to do for myself, because I love me.

You see, the devil doesn't want me to like myself. He loves it when I put myself down. When I eat too many bad things and make myself sick, the enemy wins. My bad choices help him to be victorious over me. Always dragging makes me suffer, especially when my energy levels plummet. I hate when he gets me down, and I talk negatively to myself. My adversary delights when I self-destruct and lose my hope, happiness, and good health.

I have found something wonderful that I want to share with you. I can overcome the enemy of my mind and defeat him every single time, if only I look to my Lord. When my negative voice tells me I can't do something, I lift my eyes toward heaven and listen for the still, small voice of my Lord. My God reminds me that I can do all things through Him. When my opponent tells me that I'm weak, my God reminds me He is my strength. When my mind highlights all of my failures, my God reminds me to put forth an effort for Him. When my self-doubts engage my fears, and make me think all hope is gone, I'm so thankful my God reminds me not to let my heart be troubled or afraid.

God wants us to serve Him by seeking Him and His ways continuously. Listening to the lies of the devil is unpleasing to God. God's voice is the only one we should heed. When we are distracted and listening to the devil, we can't pray or serve God, especially when we are beating ourselves into the ground with self-doubts. We can't show anyone our faith in God if we're always a nervous wreck—plagued and paralyzed with fear.

We have to rise above our fears, doubts, faults, and failures. The only way to succeed is to do the best we can, and trust that the Lord will do the rest. God wants us to speak kindly to ourselves, forgive our faults and failures, and pick up our cross and follow Him. We need to remember that we're human and will always fail and come short, but the great I AM will never fail us. After all, we love God because He first loved us. If He loves us, faults and all, and He certainly knows all about us, then we should definitely love ourselves, too.

God is always victorious. Sometimes we give up too easily and accept defeat, when in turn, we should be fighting against it. Life will never be easy. It will always be filled with challenges and hardships; however, we can overcome every single one of them through God.

We need to recognize the things bothering us and decide how to handle them. Some troubles are self-made. The enemy lies and makes things seem so much worse than they actually are. Nothing is ever as bad as the devil makes it seem. Confusion and worry distract us from our goals and lessen our joy.

When I feel overwhelmed and defeated, I pray. Regardless of what I'm going through, I have hope that either 1) it will get better, or 2) God will show me how to adapt and live through the situation. I don't think it is God's will that any type of hardship defeat me. God wants me to live every day to the fullest and fight to the very end of my life with hope always alive in my heart.

    We can all be productive and change our lives for the better. No life is worthless or hopeless. We all have daily choices, both good and bad. I am determined to focus on the good—despite my circumstances.

Despite Your Circumstances

Do you desire to make changes in your life? Have you lost your determination and zeal for God? List five things burdening your life right now and describe how you can work toward changing those hindrances. What is your determination and motivation to overcome these hindrances?

1.

2.

3.

4.

5.

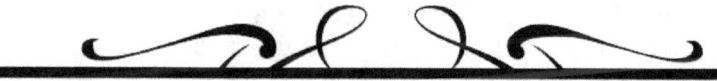

2
Eye of Faith

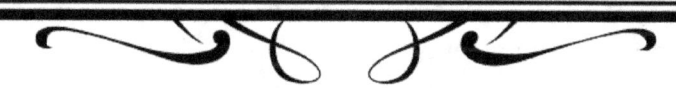

Now faith is the substance of things hoped for, the evidence of things not seen.
                              Hebrews 11:1

Faith is powerful! When exercised, it has the ability to convert the impossible into the possible. True undefiled faith has the ability to conquer the grandest mountain and endure the deepest valley. Our beliefs change our ways of thinking and show us there is more to life than we even realize.

When I think of how small I am, compared to the greatness of God and the diversity of the world, it overwhelms me. I often wonder why it is so easy to believe the bad things. It is as if my mind is programmed to listen to my negative voice, always assuming the absolute worst. I tend to believe in failure versus the realm of possibility that I can succeed. Why? Because failure takes no effort at all. It doesn't challenge me or ask that I prove myself. I can settle for whatever is comfortable and takes the least effort. In my comfort zone, everything is black and white, with no array of colors.

When everything is going great in my life, I forget about God and neglect to be thankful. I don't pray and read my Bible like I should, nor do I desire to grow in the grace and knowledge of my Lord. During the good times, faith is not needed or desired. It is in the midst of adversity and trouble that I learn the most about faith.

My God always appears in the deep recesses of the valley and proves His love to me. It amazes me, when I get to the end of my strength and God takes over. I have to fully realize my vulnerability before God will show me the grandeur of His strength.

For as long as I can remember, I have begged for the healing of my body. Being weak and challenged in my health has always burdened my life. Hardships and constant obstacles were never incorporated into the life I had envisioned for myself. As a little girl I prayed for God to heal me. These prayers continued throughout my life and into adulthood. And these prayers were not quick repetitions or without heartache. So often, I would lie in bed at night and cry myself to sleep. The pain would overwhelm me, and I didn't know how to overcome it and live my life. I never wanted to be a bitter, angry person who became hateful to everyone. Relying on others to help me was heartbreaking, and even worse was becoming their burden. It was hard for me to understand why God didn't answer my prayers. If I'm being honest, I often wondered if He loved me as much everyone around me. When we hear testimonies of how He healed other people, it's hard to understand why He didn't give us the same blessings.

Then one day, God revealed the mystery to me. *My life is not just about me!* God created me for *His* purpose. The physical healing of my scars was not part of His plan for me. God, however, will help heal the emotional pain my scars have caused. My scars and the heartaches they created have a reason. Without any pain or hardships, I wouldn't have anything to overcome. If my life was perfect, God would never enter my mind. As it is, I need Him every moment of each day.

Some days I can barely walk, sometimes my rib dislocates, and other days my hands won't work. It would be easy for me to give up and claim that all of my tasks are unattainable. My heart, however, begs to differ.

I never know what each day will hold. When I schedule events, I do so by faith. I don't know how I will feel that day. Every morning as I slide to the edge of the bed, I don't know whether I will be able to stand without pain or walk without falling. As I reach for my coffee cup, I don't know if my hand will be able to hold it. When I read my book in front of hundreds of kids, I don't know whether my rib will stay in place or whether I will struggle for each breath. Nevertheless, God will always help me. He doesn't want my excuses for why I believe I can't do these things. He wants me to keep my eyes on Him and know that He will do it for me. I just need to trust.

For me, faith is putting my life wholeheartedly into the Lord's hands. Faith is about believing in Him and His power to see me through every obstacle. He will always arrive right on time and help me overcome my troubles. God will always do what is best for me—even if it seems to hurt me in the process. Faith is about standing on the promises of the Lord.

When a new obstacle arises in my health, I know that it is something else I will have to learn to overcome. But God never puts it all on me at one time. He gives me time to adjust and learn to deal with one problem before another one occurs. With each one, we learn to trust God more and He increases our faith.

Faith demands that we listen to our hearts and ignore the rationalizations of our minds. Our beliefs are stoked by the Holy Spirit and proven by God. Faith demands that we keep our eyes on our Father. Trusting in Him doesn't allow any room for doubt. Standing among two opinions will not work. We are either a believer or an unbeliever.

As long as we doubt—about anything—we are of no help to anyone else. We open the door for the devil and give him a personal invitation to torment us. And that is like saying, *God, I really don't think You can take care of me.*

The day before one of my first school visits, I received a confirmation text: *Are you still coming tomorrow?* At that moment, my legs were numb, and walking was extremely difficult. All the reasons I couldn't go surfaced as I typed my reply. But this was what I said: *Absolutely! I can't wait!*

When we stand, feet planted firmly, not wavering at all, faith is exhibited. When the storms of life rage all around us, our hearts praise God despite the conditions. Our eyes continuously look for the blessings that God has bestowed upon us. Faith teaches us to discard negative thoughts and look for the good. Over time, we learn to take our heartaches to God and leave them on the altar at His feet.

God loves us far more than we can even imagine; He proves His love for me daily and He will do the same for you.

It has been during the darkest times of my life that I realized God's unconditional love for me. Without suffering and weakness in my body, my spirit would never have strengthened or developed such a close relationship with Him. When the realization emerges that I am nothing, I can truly see the greatness of my Lord. After all of my efforts fail and it appears there is no way, God shows me the way is by and through Him.

I'm learning to handle life with prayer and faith. There will always be obstacles to overcome, challenges to face, situations that need modifications, and heartaches to bear. When I cry out to my Lord with a broken heart, believing He will take care of it all—He does. It may not be in the way I intended, but God's ways are always the best. True faith is praising Him even before He answers our prayers. I'm learning to praise Him every day for the prayers I know He will answer.

We don't always understand the circumstances in our lives, but they do have a reason. Even when it appears that God is nowhere around, He is there. He might not always step in and prevent us from being hurt or afraid, but He can certainly soothe our heartaches and comfort our hearts.

A wonderful example can be found in the book of Daniel in the Bible. God didn't prevent Shadrach, Meshach, and Abednego from going into the fiery furnace, but He was with them the whole time. It is so important for me to remember that God is with me always. Sometimes our trials are not only just for us. They may also give others a glimpse of our God and the love He has for His children.

Despite Your Circumstances

Imagine if Shadrach, Meshach, and Abednego had whined and cried about their situation. How would that have looked to the ones gathered around them watching? We can't show anyone our faith if we are always complaining about our hardships. In all reality, we should always praise our God—regardless of whether or not our situation turns out like we wanted it to. Even when we are disobedient, God still helps us through our trials. Nothing can separate us from Him.

Exercising my faith is a lot like exercising my body. The more I do it, the easier it is to believe in the results. It is a wonderful, peaceful feeling to leave our troubles with God and not worry about them anymore. I will continue to grow my faith—despite my circumstances.

Do you ever use your faith? Are you able to praise God for the prayers and situations you know He will answer and amend? Make a list of things troubling your heart right now. Do you think God will take care of them for you? For each one, write a declaration of faith that He will.

1.

2.

3.

4.

5.

Despite Your Circumstances

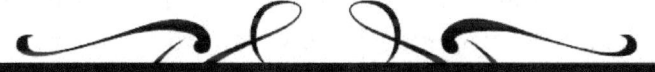

3
Positive Versus Negative

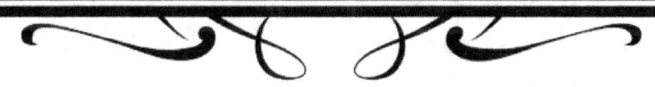

For I know the thoughts that I think toward you, saith the LORD, thoughts of peace, and not of evil, to give you an expected end.
                                        Jeremiah 29:11

The secret to happiness is really all in our head. Our joy is simply the difference between positive and negative thoughts. It is a decision we must all make. We all have the freedom of choice and are ultimately allowed to decide which one dictates our life. Every day is filled with decisions and obstacles. Some are easy while others teeter toward the edge of impossible. If you've ever encountered any hardships at all, then you know that giving up is often the easier choice. Defeat doesn't cause anyone to dig deep inside. I don't believe God can use someone who is always ready to quit. I remember the day my daddy told me, "You might as well stop trying to quit and get in there and fight."

I have often thought about my dad's words and their meaning. Did I really want to just hand the devil the victory? What if David had listened to the voice of Goliath and ignored the voice of His Lord? The odds were stacked unfavorably against him. In all reality, his situation seemed hopeless. It appeared to everyone that Goliath would kill David as he had so many others. And yet, David went in the name of the Lord. Not only did he kill the giant, but he did it with Goliath's own sword. God provides the victory!

I believe David stepped out in faith, knowing God would take care of him and make him victorious. He even praised God before the victory was ever received. If all we can see is the nemesis before us, we will forget the powerful One who lives inside us. While we can't control the things that happen to us, we can control how we handle the situation. It's all about perspective!

So often, I use the words *have to* in my daily life.

    ** I *have to* go to the grocery store.

    ** I *have to* go to the gym.

    ** I *have to* go to work.

    ** I *have to* cook dinner for my family.

    ** I *have to* go to read my kids a bedtime story.

    ** I *have to* pay bills.

    ** I *have to* help my kids with their homework.

I rarely say I "get to." However, when I change that single word, it totally changes how I feel about the statement. "Have to" sounds like a chore or a heartache, while "get to" resonates a blessing. Even my voice and facial expression differs when I make the two statements. I smile when I "get to" do something.

If we're not careful, the enemy will put our blessings in the same category as our heartaches. He is so tricky and can actually take the good things in our lives and make them seem bad. In every moment, there is something good. We just have to train our minds to search for it.

The only time bad thoughts or cruel words can hurt us is when we believe them. For example, I am frequently plagued with pain. On the good days it only last a few hours, but during the bad periods the chronic pain lasts for months. Sometimes I can still function, and then there are times when it overwhelms my mind and becomes unbearable. It would be easy for me to take medication to control the pain and my life, but I can't bear that option. The doctors have given me numerable diagnoses, all of which are incurable and debilitating. Their conclusions are filled with limitations and hopelessness, but I ignore all negativity. Don't give me limitations; give me possibilities! My abilities certainly outnumber my disabilities on any given day, but only if they are recognized. As long as we focus on the bad, then that is all we will see.

The difference between a good day and a bad day is simply our choice. Once we decide on our attitude, every other part of our day will follow. We should constantly search for the bright side of every moment. Nothing is ever as bad as it seems.

I can control my pain and mood (to some extent) in my mind. Yesterday, I was focused and determined to work all day, pain free. The week prior didn't go as well. When the alarm sounded, I made myself get up immediately. Right away the negative thoughts surrounded me. I dismissed them one by one and replaced them with positive thoughts.

> NEGATIVE VOICE: *I don't want to get up. I'm tired. My body hurts. I will never be able to do anything today. I'm just not ready to face this day and my to-do list. I hate Mondays. Is it Friday yet? I'm ready for the weekend.*

> POSITIVE VOICE: *Thank You, Lord, for waking me up and giving me another day. Thank You for helping me overcome my pain and for the ability to do the things that need to be done. I love working and I hope that You will bless me to continue. I'm thankful for every day You give me.*

Once my positive thoughts were established, I made myself eat healthy, exercise, and take my vitamins. I spent extra time on my appearance and smiled through my morning routine and the remainder of the day. When the pain and fatigue beckoned to me, I ignored them and reaffirmed my happy, positive thoughts.

> NEGATIVE VOICE: *I'm hurting. This pain is unbearable. I need to go to bed. I can't do this. I can't work today. I'm disabled. Why, God? I'm weak. I'm defeated.*

> POSITIVE VOICE: *I feel great! I'm healthy. I'm well. I'm so thankful to have a job and for all of the things I am able to accomplish each day. God is so good. I am weak, but He is strong. He will not allow me to be defeated.*

I was able to fight off the negative thoughts all day and work without any medication or tears. At the end of the day, I felt amazing. This boosted my confidence and reassured me that I'm capable of so much more than I realized. We never know our true strength until we reach our weakest moments.

One morning I woke up with my rib dislocated and my neck strained. The displacement affects my breathing and emotions. When it moves out of its normal position, it feels like everything on the right side of my body has shifted. My arm feels heavy, and I struggle to get a good, deep breath. All of these things combined make me want to cry. Sometimes tears slip out of my eyes despite my effort to hold them inside. I also get a knot in my back where the rib has shifted, and it aches continuously. Needless to say, I felt defeated. I went over my to-do list for the day and cringed at all of the things I wouldn't be able to accomplish. Right away the negative voice beckoned to me, and I ignored it. Then I gave myself a pep talk.

> *Are you always going to allow obstacles to defeat you? Don't give in to the pain! Keep going! Just put one foot in front of the other. You can do this! You're stronger than you realize. Smile and show the devil that not only can you walk, but you can run, too.*

All the while, I was lacing up my shoes. My rib hurt whether I moved or not, so I went for a run/walk. When the alarm beeped, I ran as hard as possible for one minute. Then it sounded again, and I walked for a minute and a half. While I was running, the tears surfaced and failure emerged, but I refused to give up. I kept putting one foot in front of the other and repeating my positive thoughts with

Despite Your Circumstances

a smile on my face. I had to make a decision: give up because it was hard and I was afraid to be defeated, or keep pushing and only accept defeat if it happened. So often, I fail because I give up, not because the task was too hard for me. I have learned it is all about my mind-set. If I believe I can do it, I usually will. My motto is to never give up, and I won't—despite my circumstances.

Have you ever tried the power of positive thinking? Make a list of negative thoughts or situations in your life and then write out the positive counterbalance for each one. Work on developing an attitude of gratitude.

1.

2.

3.

4.

5.

Despite Your Circumstances

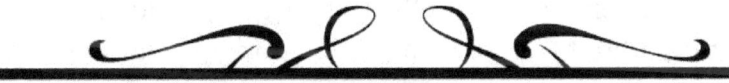

4
Overcoming Stress

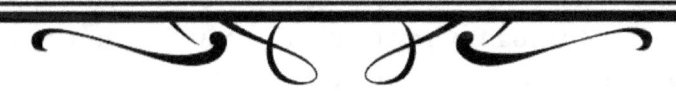

> *Peace I leave with you, my peace I give unto you: not as the world giveth, give I unto you. Let not your heart be troubled, neither let it be afraid.*
> John 14:27

Dealing with stress is one of my biggest challenges. The effect it has on my body causes me discomfort and often steals my sleep. My everyday life is filled with pressures that are overwhelming. The results of a stressful day range from minor to severe. Stress itself is not our problem. It is how we manage and deal with it that causes our trouble.

Not all stress is bad, but our body doesn't know the difference. It responds the same to both good and bad stress. The secret is finding a way to calm the tension.

Despite Your Circumstances

Things will happen beyond our control and annoy us. Loud noises will be distracting. Even the best kids occasionally throw temper tantrums. Life has a way of throwing curve balls at the worst times possible and knocking us off balance.

My life *always* seems to need some type of modification, and my goal is to focus more on solutions and less on problems. When a new deadline surfaces, right away I start finding other ways to increase the pressure in my life. If I have two weeks to accomplish a new goal, suddenly I start thinking about all of the other things that need my attention. How can I concentrate on the goal, when my toilets need to be cleaned and I have dirty windows? This self-induced frenzy makes me laugh now, but at the time I'm serious and cause myself unnecessary anxiety. Before the deadline surfaced, I wasn't even thinking about dirty windows. That is just the devil's way of distracting me. I'm learning to recognize my dramatic thoughts and stop them before they take control of me. Once I realize what is happening, it is easier to gain control and laugh at my ridiculous behavior.

Always being late is another huge, unnecessary strain in our daily lives. If I get up in plenty of time to exercise, enjoy my morning coffee with God, pray, and meditate on the commute to work, then I'm happier all day. My morning sets the tone for the rest of the day. It also makes me more pleasant to be around. No one wants to be surrounded by someone who is edgy and ready to explode in an instant.

Rushing causes our heartbeats to accelerate and our minds to race. If I wake up late and hurry to get ready, then drive fast on the way to work, I may have road rage and become irritable. Getting upset and going into crazy mode only hurts me. What helps me, however, is to change my thoughts. For example, when I'm stuck in traffic, I have learned to pray. Perhaps God halted my journey for a few moments to keep me out of harm's way. Whether I'm panicking or relaxing doesn't change the duration, but it does change the way I use my time.

Procrastination is one of the worst triggers of stress. Always waiting until the last minute is a recipe for disaster. The best technique for me is to take care of the situation immediately. When I complete my task efficiently, it also boosts my mood and gives me a sense of accomplishment. The longer I wait, the harder it is on me.

To-do lists have become my best friends. While my coffee is brewing, I start making my list of chores for the day. I break the demands down into three categories: today, tomorrow, and someday. It feels wonderful to check off my items and see how many things I have completed each day. I don't overload each day and make my list impossible to finish. That's why I make three separate lists and add to or remove things daily. Being specific is important. If I put "finish my book" on my to-do list, then I will feel overwhelmed. Writing out each individual goal (i.e., "write one page in my book"), however, helps me become more productive. Looking over my list also improves my vision of what needs to be done, and aids me in sorting my chores into the proper categories. Deadlines are not nearly as stressful as I make them out to be. Instead of viewing them as bad, I now see them as a way for me to be productive. Goals force me to get more accomplished. Those accomplishments, in turn, boost my mood and self-esteem and reduce my stress responses.

Despite Your Circumstances

Changing my views on certain things has also helped me. We don't always have to be available for everyone. In times of trouble for others, we should definitely strive to help. On the other hand, when we have deadlines and a huge to-do list, we shouldn't ignore our chores and chat with someone on the phone for hours about nothing. The same is true for instant messaging. If we're not careful, we can get caught up in the web of social media and not get anything else done. Messages, e-mails, and texts are all part of my day. Social media is an outlet that tries to steal my time. Communicating with my friends and family is great, but it has to be done in moderation. Everything needs limits, and I'm working on mine. Sometimes we just need to turn our phones off and relax. We need to step away from the *world* creating our tension.

Playing with my children, hearing them laugh, and receiving their hugs is a wonderful stress reliever. They make everything simple. Taking a walk together and skipping a little melts the fatigue and revives my spirits. Have you ever tried to skip and not smile? For me, it's impossible. My kids are wonderful blessings, and I never want to view them as heartaches or distractions. Sometimes I am pulled in so many directions that it is hard for me to balance my career, help my kids with homework, care for the home, and be a good mom. But I never want my children to be the ones to suffer. Lately, it has been trial and error for me. Giving the kids chores and explaining my situation has helped tremendously. They are learning the value of hard work and have come to understand that deadlines and heartaches are only temporal.

While I love my children dearly, they can also contribute to stress if I allow it. Families need balance, and a hectic schedule can turn them upside down. Yes, I want my children to be involved in the activities they are interested in; however, I also want to teach them the importance of family. Always running here and there, grabbing dinner at fast-food restaurants, and eating in the car is not a good way to build relationships. Regardless of what is going on in my life, my family and I always have dinner together. We may have to eat early or late, but we always manage to sit down together for a few minutes each day. Always rushing and telling them to hurry causes anxiety. It may not show up right away, but the nervous tension builds inside of everyone involved. We all need time to relax and unwind from our day. When we take on more than we can handle, some other part of our life suffers. I'm learning to schedule my days according to my needs and those of my family. Spending quality time with my family, however, is not negotiable.

Writing often helps me put things into perspective. Just a few moments with a pen and a piece of paper makes all the difference in the world. Recording my heartaches, fears, and goals improves my ability to overcome them. Usually the answer, or at least a stepping-stone toward the solution, always emerges when I write if I open my heart and become honest with myself. In addition, talking with a friend about my dilemma makes it easier for me to see the big picture and to visualize the situation outside of the box. Best friends can regularly point out our flaws, in a loving way, and help us to get back on track. We need someone who will tell us the truth without sugarcoating the facts.

Another great stress reliever is visual imagery. Spending a few moments enjoying God's beautiful masterpiece called nature improves my mood. Sunrises and sunsets are my favorite. If we can't go outdoors and take advantage of the moments, pictures work as well. Looking at a beautiful ocean scene dissolves my tension. It causes me to breathe deeply and become more relaxed. For a moment, I find myself inside the image, happy and content. When I truly focus on being there, the moment becomes more real. I can feel the sun and breeze, smell the salt water, hear the waves crashing on the beach, and touch the sand. Visual imagery works the same for my goals and dreams. When the writing process becomes overwhelming and it seems impossible to finish my book, I imagine holding it in my hands. In my mind, there are kids surrounding me, all smiling as I read my new story to them. I see them enjoying the coloring sheets and the characters. I envision whom the book is designed for and get a clear picture in my head. When I want to stop and give up, the picture surfaces and God reminds me of my purpose.

Prayer is the best medicine for a troubled soul. When I spend time alone with my heavenly Father, the passion I have for Him melts away all stress. I love to mediate on His Word. In fact, meditation is a wonderful way to relax and get rid of the tension in our bodies. Once a day, I take a few moments to overcome the stressors of my day and refocus with positive thoughts and encouraging scriptures.

Good things can also cause our bodies to feel tension. When my books were released, there were so many great things happening that I couldn't sleep. As a result, my shoulders tensed and caused pain in my neck, and I experienced headaches and a nervous stomach. Too much excitement can hurt us. That's why it is so important to rid ourselves of nervous tension. It's kind of like kids who have so much energy that they need to play, run, and burn some of it off. We reach that point, as well. Exercise is a huge part of de-stressing my life, and it provides a release of tension regardless of the source. It not only causes endorphins to be released in our bodies, but it also promotes better sleep.

We all must learn to conquer the stressors of our lives. I have decided to be an overcomer—despite my circumstances.

Despite Your Circumstances

Do you handle your stress successfully or do you allow it to control you? What are some ways that you cope with the daily stressors of life?

1.

2.

3.

4.

5.

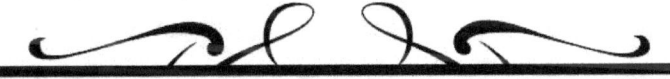

5
A Mile in My Shoes

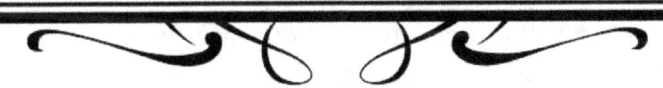

The LORD is my strength and my shield; my heart trusted in him, and I am helped: therefore my heart greatly rejoiceth; and with my song will I praise him.

Psalm 28:7

We never know what the road ahead will be like. We don't know how many bumps, turns, valleys or steep mountains we will endure. Regardless of the terrain or weather, however, most of us will never take a single step without guidance and strength from God. Even when we can't feel Him or hear Him, He is there. He is ever-present—loving and merciful, with grace for every need.

Despite Your Circumstances

Today, I caught a glimpse of the person I used to be. At the playground with my children, I noticed a child in the shadows who was not interacting with the others. I could tell by her wistful expression that she wanted to play, as well, but for whatever reason, she held back. For a moment, I watched her and remembered. Once upon a time, the shy little girl alone in the corner of the playground was me. My heart recalled being the invisible girl whom all the others walked right by. The image took me back to the times when I tried to hide my scars and dreamed of just being normal. I was the one who was afraid to make friends, the one who thought no one could possibly befriend me.

Then I witnessed a wonderful transformation. Someone walked over and asked the child to play, and her whole demeanor changed. Suddenly, it no longer mattered to anyone that she was different—even in her own thoughts. The children laughed and played, and for a few moments, in their world, differences simply didn't matter and everyone was the same.

Fear is the absolute worst part about being different. The unknown is the hardest part to overcome. Not knowing how others will receive us is often the reason we never venture out. No one wants to be rejected or teased, or always be the spotlight of the moment. Hesitation and doubts prevent us all, at some point in our lives, from moving forward in the direction our hearts desire to go. It is easier to believe the worst-case scenario than it is to consider that good things might happen. We need to train ourselves to understand that with God all things are possible, and then we must do our best to make sure others know, as well.

Children are so much stronger than we give them credit for. I've witnessed a few who are far stronger than I will ever be. Some go through life without enough kindness, encouragement, praise, discipline, or love. As bad as all that sounds, positive and hopeful things can still emerge out of the bad situations.

We can help those struggling by giving them hope and encouragement and by showing them that God will work it all out. Through my own life, I want to reassure others that God will turn their heartaches into blessings. Our struggles and triumphs might be their window into a better day, or perhaps their light during the darkest of times. God can use us to give them encouragement when the road seems impossible, or to help them when they feel overwhelmed. Our story may offer hope when it seems all hope is gone, and give them testimony and proof that God has a purpose for each life.

At some point we all have walked a mile in their shoes, and experienced hurtful, awful, and bleak situations. If we search our minds, we can recall these times and how the hopelessness of it all bombarded our lives. I remember the bellyaches and tears in the bathroom between classes, the continuous prayers and desire for God to make it all better, holding it all inside of me and not wanting anyone to know I was hurting so bad. It is extremely difficult for us all to bare our souls and ask for support. No one ever wants to be the person who is scarred, affected by trauma, abused, neglected, or abandoned. We all want the perfect life, with no heartaches, trials, or problems of any kind. Unfortunately, no one goes through life without some hardships. So often I wished for someone who would understand my pain and be able to help me—without me having to admit my heartaches. We need to be an example of hope to these people. Perhaps that's why I want to walk an extra mile to make a difference.

My heart embraces the incredible vision that I can make a difference in someone's world. God has blessed me and my story to touch so many lives. He purposed each life before we were even born, and He will bring His purpose to pass. We can help these children and adults alike who struggle in their lives.

I started writing to be heard and not seen. I wanted to cowardly hide behind my scars. It was my intention to help others but never experience any personal growth or change myself. Thankfully, God had other plans.

The first time someone contacted me and wanted to conduct an interview, I cried—not tears of joy or thankfulness, but tears of sorrow and ultimate fear. Interviews were never part of the writer's life or fantasy, I had assumed. It never occurred to me that anyone would ever want to write an article about me. The fear of what they would say almost paralyzed me. I had no idea this would come with being published. Had I known, it would have been extremely hard to sign my contracts. Today, I'm thankful that ignorance is often bliss.

Sometimes when we start on a journey, we have no idea all of the rough terrain we will be forced to endure. If we knew all of the bumps and bruises and twists and falls we would experience, then we would never be able to take a single step forward. God fixes it so that we only encounter a little at a time, and then He helps us to overcome each one. Every time He brings me through the impossible, it creates a memory of triumph for me. Then the next time a similar obstacle occurs, I can pull up the memory and focus on how He delivered me out of the enemy's hand.

The transformation God performed in me is miraculous and amazing. Only God has the power to transform a shy little girl who often shoved her hands in her pockets and who refused to wear open-toed shoes and sleeveless shirts, into a positive, thankful person. God is the only One with enough peace to calm the fear inside me, and evoke the courage needed to speak at conferences, do book signings, appear on television, and visit schools. Now I'm able to talk about my scars and help others who are struggling. It is God who gives me the bravery to open my heart and allow others to glimpse the person underneath it all. One of the greatest and most unexpected blessings is the way other people see me. People have told me they never saw my scars because of my smile.

The one thing I have learned is that everyone has some type of hardship to overcome. When I read one of my Zippy books to a group of kids, they all relate to his story. They all feel the connection of being different, of sometimes being left out or feeling insecure.

When I speak to group of adults, they all nod their heads or wipe tears from their eyes. We have all walked the same path, just in different ways. Sometimes we need to be reminded that we are not alone. It is my goal to be more considerate of others, and to strive to make a difference every single day in someone's life. Our lives would be better if we would all adhere to the Golden Rule and love everyone as ourselves.

The first step in our journey starts with kindness. It's contagious. Walk a mile with me and help me to spread it around—despite your circumstances.

Despite Your Circumstances

Is there a desire inside you to make a difference? What could you do to help your community and loved ones? Make a list and commit to it.

1.

2.

3.

4.

5.

6
God's Creativity

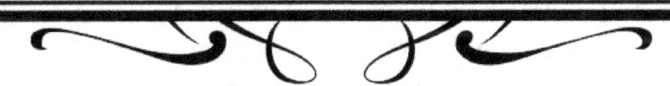

Even every one that is called by my name: for I have created him for my glory, I have formed him; yea, I have made him.

Isaiah 43:7

It's so easy to forget that God created us all. He has had His hands on us with every step. There were no mistakes or accidents that occurred. He looked through time and saw a need for each life He created. And so He designed each person according to that need. Of course, we all like to be critical of His work. We like to complain about our features and even try to change them. What we often forget is that the person underneath can triumph over the shell of their body. But as long as the devil can make us focus on our imperfections, he has us distracted.

For example, if someone laughed and made fun of our teeth or called us ugly, it would be difficult for us to talk and smile. Our natural reaction would be to hide our imperfections. In doing so, we would miss out on many opportunities and suppress the wonderful person inside of us all. It doesn't matter what we look like on the surface, when we smile, our faces become beautiful because they glow from the inside out. The outward appearance is just a vessel to hold the beautiful gift God gave us.

It makes us all feel bad about ourselves when someone tells us we're overweight, handicapped, or broken. Negative comments attack our self-esteem and confidence. Harsh words have a way of lingering in our minds and overpowering any compliments.

The world cannot see our *true* beauty. The part that shines so brightly is hidden deep inside, beneath layers of scars and dust. It is our responsibility to give that part of ourselves a little glimpse every now and then. We can only let our true beauty out when we accept ourselves.

I guess I'm a good one to talk about acceptance—the girl who prayed every night for God to heal her hands. Before God would allow me to share my books and the beautiful testimony of my life, I had to accept my scars completely. Right before it all happened, it was as if God asked me a question: *Do you still want Me to heal your hands?* I knew I had to make a choice: to have beautiful, unscarred hands, or to accept my scars along with everything else God purposed just for me. It wasn't a decision of my mind, but my heart. For a moment, I wanted to allow God to take my scars away. But in the next instant, I was so relieved and thankful that He never answered my prayer. God knew His purpose for me was far greater than any heartache I would ever encounter.

The Master had compassion on me when He intervened and spared me in my mother's womb. He understood that I would hate being scarred and realize that people would stare, treat me badly, tease, bully, and break my heart on many occasions. My Creator saw that I was destined for a life of struggles and prejudice, but He also saw the day of my complete acceptance and thankfulness. God looked beyond the heartache, trials, and tribulations, and He envisioned a greater purpose than my simply being unscarred. When He looked at me, there was no glimpse of a burdened life, but instead He saw a window to Himself.

My scars were not created for punishment, but for His glory. Hands that appear broken, but have amazing abilities, provide a glimpse of Him. When they ache and swell, but still manage to tuck sweet little boys in at night, wash dishes, prepare meals, clean the house, do the laundry, drive, carry burdens, show love, turn pages in books, and help others, it touches people and gives them hope.

God gives me just enough heartache and struggles to keep me grounded. He also provides adequate strength and determination to help me persevere. I believe it was difficult for Him when He lifted me out of the entanglement of the bands and purposed that I would be scarred. And yet, my Lord created me with love (as He did with everyone) and made it so that I would be blessed.

Loving arms patiently awaited my birth. God specifically awarded me with the most wonderful parents, who may not have chosen my scars, but who loved me despite my challenges and accepted every part of me. They never made excuses for me or treated me any differently from my siblings. My parents surrounded me with love and always boosted my confidence. In fact, they handled my scars so well that I wondered at times if they could even see that I was different.

All through my life, the Lord gave me so many amazing people to love and accept me. God provided a solid foundation for me to grow and develop into the person He created me to be. He taught me how to weather the storms and rise above my circumstances. Many times He placed me in the fire to mold me into a stronger person for Him and guide me deeper along on my quest.

Sometimes we give up on our lives and think we are finished, when we still have so much we could do. We make our lives all about us, when it should be about our God. It's hard to focus on our purpose when we are so self-absorbed in what we want for ourselves. In order to be a mighty vessel for God, we have to give our lives back to Him and allow Him to use us as He sees fit.

We all have talents. God didn't slight anyone. The difference is simply that some people use their God-given talents, while others waste their lives. This may seem harsh, but it's true. The only way to fully use our lives and capabilities is through God. Every day we should ask God these simple questions: *What can I do for You today? How can I use my talent for Your honor and glory?* When I focus on helping others, my heartaches and problems don't seem as bad.

God creates us all with purpose and prospers us with love. I will be the person I was created to be—despite my circumstances.

Have you ever thought about your God-given purpose? Do you feel you are living the life God created you to live? Make a list of ways you currently use or want to use your special gift(s) for God.

1.

2.

3.

4.

5.

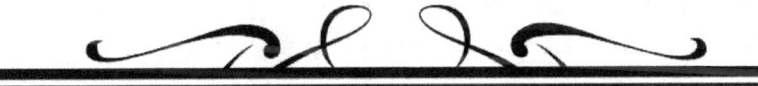

7
Making a Difference

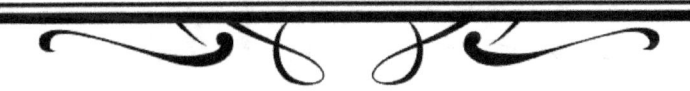

When a man's ways please the LORD, he maketh even his enemies to be at peace with him.
                                    Proverbs 16:7

Not everyone will like us. Regardless of what we do or how much we try, someone will always find fault with us. It has nothing to do with our scars, weight, beauty, accomplishments, failures, or wealth. It is usually the result of jealousy and bitterness. It is a form of evil that lurks in us all.

I have been both the bully and the one who was bullied. We all have. There are times in our lives when we all succumb to the darkness inside of us. We forget that kindness is not the absence of hatred; it's the overcoming of it. We have to train ourselves to act accordingly. We have to decide what type of person we want to be and then strive to achieve it.

I cannot control how other people treat me, but I can decide my own behavior and the way I treat others. We will not find any excuse anywhere to be mean to another soul. The ones who treat us the worst in life are the ones who need our love and kindness the most. They require us to talk to the Lord on their behalf. Despite their actions, they desire our prayers, love, and hope. If we follow our hearts and cry out to God, we could possibly be a lighthouse during their storm.

We have all glimpsed the eyes of a troubled soul. It is not forgettable to encounter someone with so much heartache that it radiates from them. The pain can be so severe that the injured will lash out, even hurting the one trying to offer comfort and assistance. It is a coping mechanism to protect themselves, however possible.

I will never forget looking down into the coffin of a lifeless child. The young girl had been in so much pain that she ended her own life. A part of me can't even imagine what that type of pain feels like, and yet, my heart understands. I have lived with torment, limitations, and numerous other obstacles. It seems like only yesterday when I cried and prayed for God to make it all stop. Being bullied hindered me from concentrating on my schoolwork. My stomach would hurt, along with my heart, and I couldn't understand how anyone could be so cruel. It was such a struggle for me to take their cruelty without retaliating. Maybe a part of it was fear of what they would do to me. The other part was compassion. I didn't want them to suffer as I had. In spite of it all, I wanted to be friends.

I don't think they realized how different life was for me. I had to keep up with my classmates and figure out how to do all of the work on my own. Very early in my life, I experienced pain in my shoulders, arms, and hands. Just carrying my books was challenging on the bad days, but I didn't want to complain because I was afraid of what would happen. I didn't want to be put in special classes because I still held on to the illusion of a normal life. So I took whatever the students and teachers dished out to me.

Not everyone was mean to me. Some kind souls influenced my life, too. Their kindness reached into my heart and healed the ache. God gave me special friends to laugh with and love. He also put great teachers in my path to encourage and motivate me. A kind word or a look of understanding helped me through my day.

Not only was I bullied in school, but I was mistreated in the workplace, as well. To this day, I don't understand why certain people treat others so badly. It is almost as if the bully tries to destroy all of another's self-worth. They seem to believe that it makes them look good when other people fail. But that couldn't be further from the truth.

When we push someone down, we are also lashing out at God. Whatever we do to others, we also do to our Lord. Jesus said, "And the King shall answer and say unto them, Verily I say unto you, inasmuch as ye have done it unto one of the least of these my brethren, ye have done it unto me" (Matthew 25:40). I cannot recall one time when the enemy successfully triumphed over God. We should think about our actions before we act, and decide who we are living for. If we are living for God, we shouldn't be mimicking the enemy. People should be able to take one look at us and see who dwells in our hearts.

I want to be involved in my children's lives. It is my job to watch their behavior and sense any changes in their persona. If there is something happening at school, it will show in their actions. I often ask questions and visit the school when time permits. Volunteering for a few hours in my children's classrooms shows me exactly what is going on, and helps me to see what I need to do as a parent. Seeing how my kids interact with others lets me know if they themselves have issues I should address.

We can stop bullying! The future generations will be educated by our words and actions. Our children need to be taught how to treat others. It's really quite simple. We need to enforce positive behavior, pay attention to our children, hug them when they need it, and discipline them when they need that, too. We must *show* them love every single day, and strive to be their role models in life. We can stop bullying.

I've heard so many parents make the comment that they can't do anything with their children. While it may seem impossible at the time, we can mold our children into what they should be. It takes love, patience, persistence, discipline, tears, and prayers, but we can do it!

Dinner was once stressful for me. My child refused to try anything new, and he was always convinced that he didn't like it. My husband and I began to enforce the one-bite rule. He had to at least try the food to see whether he liked it or not. That one bite would sometimes take an hour to complete. There would be tears and gagging, screaming, and the most ridiculous behavior possible. Many times, I wanted to give up, but I didn't. Our son eventually realized that his temper tantrums wouldn't get him his way. It would, however, cause him trouble. So he eventually complied with our rules, and a wonderful thing happened. Once the fits ceased, he discovered many new foods that he liked.

If we allow our children to intimidate us, then they will treat others the same way. It may not seem that important, but our words and actions do affect our children. We may think they're not listening, but when it counts they will be reminded of our words. When I was a child, my mom always encouraged me. She would always tell me, "Find your own way, Candida. You can do anything." During hard times, when I felt like giving up, I could hear her encouraging words. They made a big difference to me.

Ever since my books were released, I have traveled to schools and shared Zippy with the students. My Zippy books give them a visual image about teasing and bullying, as well as the emotions and feelings attached to these actions. After reading my book, I speak out about bullying and encourage the children to dream and believe in themselves.

One day God blessed me with the opportunity to speak to one of the biggest bullies in the school. He used Zippy and me to paint a vivid picture of what bullying does to another soul. Together we reached that child—I saw the transformation in his demeanor and the tears in his eyes.

At another school, a child ran up to her teacher after my presentation and apologized for her bad behavior. She had been in trouble just that morning for bullying another child. I believe deep down, in the recesses of my heart, that Zippy and I can make a difference.

Despite Your Circumstances

Sometimes all we need to do is try. We need to stand up for these children, as well as for ourselves. It takes effort, but we can reach the unreachable. Through kindness, we can touch everyone and show them friendship. In doing so, we can offer them a glimpse of God. Our passion for life may inspire and offer hope to those who have lost it all.

I love to volunteer and give from my heart. We sometimes feel our contributions, big or small, will not change anything, but it might. Hope and effort are the things that alter the world. Compliments and encouragement can go a long way to brighten someone else's day. Reading a book about bullying and how to overcome it to a classroom may not only help the children being bullied, but it may also help the bullies realize the effects of their actions.

Sometimes we tend to make excuses for our bad behavior, instead of looking for ways to become a better person. I hear so many excuses and have made many of my own. Any type of accomplishment usually takes sweat, heartache, sacrifices, determination, prayers, and love to obtain. The things in life that are the hardest for us to achieve are usually the most worthwhile.

Life is not always easy for me. Some nights I lay awake, battered with sickness and nerves. The enemy always tries to stop me and place nearly impossible obstacles in my way. If fear won't stop me, then he resorts to illness. One morning I was so sick, I gagged with every nibble of cracker. My stomach heaved and my palms sweated. It would have been so easy for me to cancel my school visit that day. After all, I had a valid excuse—being terribly sick. God, however, gave me the determination to see it through. He held my hand the whole time and helped me to see the devil's tricks and even overcome them. Through prayer and positive thinking, I was able to complete the school visit. In an unexplainable way, God prevailed and rewarded me for my effort. He also gave me a moment of triumph to record. If we declare something to be too hard or not possible, we deceive ourselves and accept failure based on a lack of effort. Our children deserve more. We need to teach, through our own lives, the possibilities of positive change.

Our world has become corrupt due in part to our actions. Now is not the time for us to throw in the towel, so to speak. It is the opportunity for us to show the beauty of hard work and dedication. We need to teach our children to always preserve and walk by faith, regardless of the trial.

If we truly tried and gave our life the grandest effort, the possibilities would amaze us all. Kindness and the ability to show God's love make a huge difference in me. We should strive to make a difference for others—despite our circumstances.

Despite Your Circumstances

List several ways you can make a difference in your world.

1.

2.

3.

4.

5.

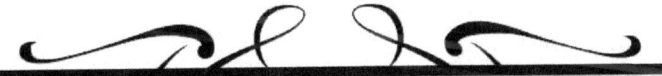

8
Testing Times

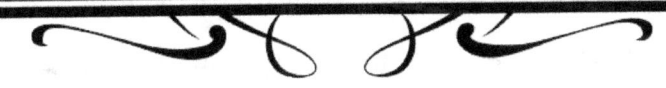

> *Beloved, think it not strange concerning the fiery trial which is to try you, as though some strange thing happened unto you: But rejoice, inasmuch as ye are partakers of Christ's sufferings; that, when his glory shall be revealed, ye may be glad also with exceeding joy.*
>
> 1 Peter 4:12–13

The world is filled with stipulations. We tend to need scientific reasoning for why things happen. People like to put things in nice, neat segments based on cause and effect, statistics, and conclusions. It is impossible for our minds to understand miracles. We want every situation to be simple or we want a lengthy explanation as to why it happened. The possibility that many aspects of life are beyond our control is not acceptable.

No one likes being referred to as a "condition" or a having bunch of statistics attached to them. But I am nothing more than a sinner saved by grace, who found mercy in the eyes of my Lord. He is the One who made me a survivor. So often, we look at our lives and all that we've had to endure, and we forget that we *survived* the trauma. We focus on the details of our ordeal and neglect to enjoy our beautiful lives. People and situations can only hurt us if we allow them to.

Sometimes we need to put our own lives into perspective. As long as we view ourselves as victims, the enemy wins. Whenever we dramatically change our lives because of events beyond our control, the evil overtakes us. If our every thought is about how we were victimized, then we allow the bad to take our lives, as well.

It doesn't matter what happened, because for some reason, God blessed us to survive. Our suffering has a reason and it is all part of God's plan for us. No condition or circumstance has the ability to destroy us. Determination and a strong will to thrive are inside of us all.

We should focus on beating the odds, and marvel at how God blesses us to do the impossible. It is wonderful to exhibit faith and follow our hearts into new territory. When we stand on the promises of the Lord and follow His ways, even when they appear to be unfathomable, the enemy is without power or control over us.

Let's face it, God doesn't ask much of anyone, and our experience is not comparable to how Jesus suffered for us. I do believe, however, that there are times when we are tested. We are given situations to see how we will react. It's the reaction to the test that shows exactly where our hearts lie.

If we give up every time life gets hard, we will never accomplish anything. It is not the number of obstacles we face, but the ones we overcome that is important. The enemy will never stop trying to take away our enjoyment of living. We should learn to use our trials as a burst of energy to prevail, instead of a burden of defeat.

Walking had become nearly impossible for me. A combination of pain, numbness, a twisted pelvis, and the malformation of my left foot threatened to halt me. Even when I managed to push through the pain, blisters formed on my foot and my knee swelled.

Comfortable, practical shoes definitely made the most sense. High heels, however, make me feel invincible. I have always loved them, even when I played in them as a little girl. When I get ready to do school visits, my appearance helps boost my confidence. It is one thing to *be* beautiful, and another to *feel* beautiful—and so I always try to wear high heels. Also, heels prevent me from limping (which I frequently do), and during school visits, I don't want to limp.

One day while standing in a store surrounded by shoes, I was distraught. Pair after pair lay discarded in the floor and defeat settled in my heart. I limped and dragged my numb leg down the aisles, as I concentrated on each pair and how they would make me feel. To be honest, I don't know how it happened, but I walked out of the store with a pair of red high heels in my hands and tears in my eyes. Through my small test that day, I learned the meaning of the phrase "Pain is inevitable, but suffering is optional."

Although wearing heels wasn't possible at the time, they represented the hope of a better day to me, and they made me feel beautiful. After all, every girl needs a pair of red high heels to kick the enemy out of her way and provide hope when everything else seems hopeless.

A few years ago, I was attending an event at my son's school when I noticed a woman with no hair. I knew she had cancer and had been battling the disease for some time. Suddenly, I felt ashamed of my long hair. There I sat with hair way down my back, while she didn't even have eyelashes. My beautiful hair that was often praised and admired by others now seemed heavy and selfish to me.

God gave me the thought to donate my hair to an organization that makes wigs for those in need. At first, my mind wasn't willing to even contemplate the thought. It was my hair, and I didn't want to cut it. I began to question how my hair could really make a difference. Even as I tried to justify my reasoning for not doing it, the burden to help others weighed heavily on my heart. And then it happened. My hair changed in my eyes. It was no longer beautiful or loved. It was a constant reminder to me that there were people who had to fight to live. If my hair could give someone a smile, encouragement to keep fighting their battle, or a little strength on their weaker days, then it would be worth it. So I made my appointment and cut off more than ten inches of my hair. God blessed me with an amazing feeling and a prayer for those suffering.

My new hairstyle was a shock, not only to me, but to everyone I saw. And God gave me a beautiful testimony to accompany it. After I donated my hair, my sister also donated hers. The generosity continued through friends and family. God's blessings are never void. They always achieve greatness.

God showed me another degree of His love through this small test. So often, we desire to help others, but when the opportunity is presented we want another option. We want to pick and choose how we extend our love and help, but God wants us to love unconditionally. He wants us to love all of His children and also to show our love. Sometimes we have to do something to affect another life and show the love of God in us. We need to be willing to do whatever God beckons us to do. There is a reason and a purpose for everything. When He burdens our heart with a task, there is a plan already in place. He knows the result from start to finish, the lives it will affect, and the hearts it will touch. Sometimes He even allows our kindness to have a boomerang effect. When we think we are too small to make a difference, we need to remember, God is God and He can do the things that are impossible for us to do.

I believe God places angels on this earth to teach us and to test our reactions. He may show us someone with scars to see whether we recognize the power of inner beauty. A handicapped person might remind us to slow down and be thankful for all that we are able to do. Blindness may very well instruct us to see with our hearts. Deafness could possibly school us on the wonders of sound. Someone stricken with disease could educate us on the quality of life.

Once during a conference, I heard a story about a man who had been badly burned. Even some of his limbs and features were lost in the fire. The person telling the story referred to him as a monster and explained how everyone was pointing, staring, and murmuring about him. He then proceeded to explain how he ended up sitting beside the man and befriending him. That's how we should all be—ready and willing to embrace the differences of others. When I heard this story, I cried for all the people who couldn't see the miracle right before their eyes, and for the man who lives every day with pain because of the cruelty of others.

No one is exempt from heartaches. Everyone has or will have burdens to bear and obstacles to overcome. We should always follow our hearts and extend kindness whenever possible. One day we could be fighting the same battles.

Life is filled with tests. Some are easy, and others are extremely difficult. We need to stop during our tests and make sure we are learning the things God is trying to teach us. If we get angry and become blind to our lessons, then we may fail the test and be forced to repeat it.

God never gives us any type of hardship without a reason. Each one is tailored to our specific needs and provides the greatest benefit for us. During the trial we may feel as if God is mad or has forsaken us, but the truth is that He wants us to be the best that we can be. He wants us to be an exceptional student and graduate to higher levels—despite our circumstances.

List some important tests in your life and the lessons you learned from them.

1.

2.

3.

4.

5.

9
Running Our Race

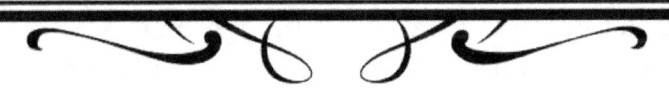

Wherefore seeing we also are compassed about with so great a cloud of witnesses, let us lay aside every weight, and the sin which doth so easily beset us, and let us run with patience the race that is set before us.

Hebrews 12:1

We are all on a journey, one filled with hardships, joy, suffering, and great victories. It takes training, the right mind-set, and determination to learn how to run our race with patience. Our victories don't happen overnight. God doesn't want us to faint when we are overwhelmed, but rather to seek Him. If we keep trying to overcome our obstacles, God will show us how to live beyond our limitations. Sometimes we have to go to the very edge of reasoning, and then take a leap of faith. We don't have to know all of the details; we only need to realize that our Lord is beside us every step of the way. He uses our hardships and sufferings to create our joy and victories.

It took me three years to run a 5K, but each step was imperative and made the victory so much greater. If I had accomplished the task immediately, then I wouldn't have learned the power of overcoming.

My son wanted to run in his school's Race for School Health: Relay for Life. He believed his effort would truly help cancer patients. Because he was under the age limit, however, he needed an adult to run with him. It broke my heart to not be by his side, but my body wasn't ready. At that point, walking was difficult for me, causing my legs go numb after only five minutes.

On race day, my little boy was so nervous that his stomach became upset. Even though he was sick, he still pushed through each mile and received a second-place award. I would like to think my example of overcoming obstacles helped him be able to conquer his own. I was so proud of him, but disappointed that I wasn't the one who ran by his side. As my sister ran with him, I vowed to be there the next year.

Months prior to the next year's race, I started my training. My foot's formation challenges my balance on one leg, as well as my ability to jump, walk, and run. The weight landing on one foot was painful during and after my training sessions. Determination kept me motivated, but the difficulty of the task stressed my body. I continued to push through the pain and prepare for the race. I checked my children's backpacks daily for the signup sheet. But then I discovered the race had already taken place. My oldest son hadn't wanted to participate, and he convinced my youngest, who did want to race, not to tell me until afterward. At first, I was furious. I had trained very hard and even suffered to be able to participate. But then, I laughed.

We all tend to make things much greater than they actually are. I had tormented myself and worried about something that was actually insignificant. All I could see was my inability to run by his side, and I forgot to factor in my influence of beating the odds. Without determination it is impossible to accomplish any task.

One morning, I couldn't decide if I wanted to cry or go back to bed. My body ached, and I couldn't seem to get past the misery. I sulked and finally dragged myself to the gym, expecting my workout to lift my spirits. My experience, however, was not what I hoped for.

My body felt heavy and uncooperative. Ignoring all negativity, I decided to run. It was hard—well, actually, it was brutal. My rib hurt, a blister developed on my foot after the first mile, and my legs were heavy. Being stubborn, I refused to give up even when my legs grew numb. So I pushed beyond my limits. And then the treadmill just stopped. I was furious. It was like the machine knew that I didn't have enough sense to step off on my own, so it just quit. Instead of stretching and leaving, I moved to the elliptical for a few miles. Every movement hurt, and I realized after two miles that I couldn't do any more. I tried to dig deep, but I had nothing left to give. Defeated, I grabbed my things and left.

At the time, I couldn't see that I had still managed three miles with numbness and tingling in my feet and legs. Then I remembered my daddy's words of wisdom: "You're doing better than what you think." Instead of feeling better, though, I dwelled on what I couldn't do. I believed what I had always assumed and been told. It was so hard for me to accept my limitations. Nevertheless, I tried. I even attempted to forgive my body for not being able to do something that I truly wanted to do. Who was I kidding? It hurt. And I didn't like the disability card. Ever!

Then, the next day, I went back to the gym for one more attempt, and I decided to try a new approach. When I set the treadmill to run the 5K, I began with a smile and praise for my Lord. As my feet pounded, I thanked God for every step, and for letting me not only walk that day, but for the ability to run. I prayed for all of those who were not able to walk and run, those who were fighting for their lives, and those who had heartaches and troubles.

When I reached the point where my whole body ached, I smiled at my reflection. I was only a mile into my run, and the screen showed that my course would get even harder. For a moment, I wanted to stop, to step off the machine and agree with the doctors and the negative voice in my head—that I couldn't run. Then I realized it was during the most challenging times in our lives that we learn how to overcome. My legs were still moving. It was my mind that wanted to give up. So I focused on how it would feel to complete my course. I'll be quite honest: I imagined every time my foot came down that I was stomping on the devil, the one who threatened to steal my hopes and dreams.

With my heart and my spirit, I finished my first 5K program. It took me forty minutes to do the impossible. While my aches and pains proved that I fought the battle, I also have the victory written in my heart. That victory will remind me on the tough days to keep my eyes on my Lord.

Last year, when walking was difficult for me, I lay in my bed and pedaled an exercise bike that sat on it. When my feet grew numb and painful, I pushed with my heart and the determination that I would get better.

The enemy will take our lives if we allow him to. We need to fight with every ounce of strength we can manage. Every day we are in the biggest battle of our lives. We get to decide what kind of solider we want to be. I want to fight a good fight. If we give up every time our course gets tough, then we will never reach our full potential.

When my son finally brought home the dreaded form for the race again, I decided to try. God had already proven to me that I could do it. On race day I was so nervous, but my family surrounded me—encouraging and supporting me.

A half a mile in, my legs went numb. They felt so heavy and painful. But while my mind wanted to stop, my body was still going. Two miles into the race, my ribs dislocated and my chest hurt. I struggled for every breath, and to be honest, I just wanted it to be over. When we rounded the corner, I felt the tears, and I had to make a decision—keep going or give up. Once I decided to keep going, the most wonderful thing happened. My sister sang the theme song for Zippy: "Be the Best That You Can Be," and God picked me up in His arms and carried me.

My sister and I both cried at the finish line, and the smile on my son's face was priceless. He was so proud of me. Although he had watched my struggles for years, he also witnessed my victory. It might have taken me three years, but God helped me run my race with patience and finish the impossible—despite my circumstances.

Despite Your Circumstances

How do you handle challenges in your life? Do you faint when you are challenged, or do you take a leap of faith and keep trying to overcome your obstacles? Make a list of encouraging phrases to help you run your race with patience and determination.

1.

2.

3.

4.

5.

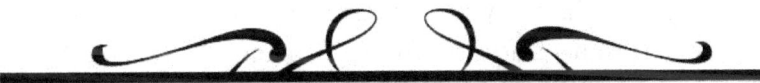

10
Our Stories

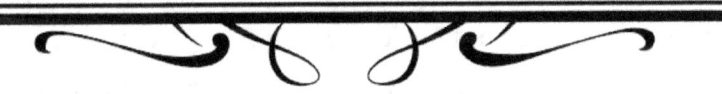

Be still, and know that I am God: I will be exalted among the heathen, I will be exalted in the earth.

Psalm 46:10

When God does something, He does it *big*, and He always makes it look so easy.

My books, which had taken me seven years to complete, were finally finished. I was so relieved and happy. I sent the manuscripts out into the publishing world with query letters accompanied by prayers. They returned to me, however, unpublished and hopeless.

I resorted to finding a literary agent to help. I remember when I finally submitted *Underneath the Scars* to one whom God had shown me would help, but instead, he rejected my manuscript and declared that it didn't have the ability to touch anyone's heart. I was devastated. I called my husband, and while sobbing into the phone I confessed that I had quit. I remember such pain and anguish in my heart. What I couldn't see at the time was that God was moving—getting His plan in order.

I decidedly laid my manuscript down at the Lord's feet. With much tears and groaning, I turned it all over to Him. I had gone as far as possible for me to go, and I knew I didn't have the power to make it happen on my own. I remember telling my family that I would just give my book away. But that wasn't a part of God's plan. Instead, He blessed my heart to write a blog. I had absolutely no clue what I was doing, but I desired to follow His leading and write the words that burdened me.

In February 2011, I published my first blog entry and established my writing career. Even though I had told God that no one would want to read my blog, I quickly developed followers all over the world. Their dedication and support gave me the confidence I needed to keep writing and dreaming.

Then one day, everything changed. I was about as low as anyone could get. Others had urged me to sign up for a disability check, and my heart was almost convinced they were right. I paced the floors after my husband went to work and my children left for school, and I prayed. I begged God to help me get better and allow me to work again. I felt helpless and so scared. My heart believed there was something good around the corner and I just needed to wait for it. I can't even explain the power of that tiny spark of hope. It held my hopes, my dreams, and my life. Regardless of the odds, there was something greater urging me to not give up. I'm sure my family thought I was being unrealistic at times, but still they supported me and my dreams. Then, out of the blue, I received an e-mail that changed my life.

I was sitting in line to pick up my kids from school, when my phone alerted me to a new e-mail. I stared at the screen in disbelief. ShadeTree Publishing had contacted me and asked whether I'd like to write books for them. I had never heard of them or submitted anything to their company before, but a mutual friend had shared my blog. They had read it and liked my writing style. Things like this don't just happen. These are God Moments.

God Moments are not predictable or even explainable. They cross boundaries and bestow something far greater than even imaginable. They are always exactly the right thing at the right time. They leave us in awe, with an unmovable smile.

I submitted *Underneath the Scars* and knew in my heart this was God moving. A few weeks later I was offered a contract and experienced the blissful moment of experiencing my dreams come true. This time my heart agreed. Sometimes we have to walk by faith and trust God. He had brought me to this moment, and I knew He would take care of me. He answered my prayers even greater than I had imagined. Not only did I receive a contract for *Underneath the Scars*, but they wanted to publish *Zippy and the Stripes of Courage*, as well. Suddenly, God was giving me not one book, but two.

Despite Your Circumstances

My little Zippy had, until then, been tucked away in a drawer and deemed hopeless. I remembered the day I cried and grieved for him and his story that would never be shared and enjoyed by children. I remembered how my heart ached when I put him away. I remembered how I had desired to go into schools to share him and make a difference in some life, somewhere.

Just when I thought it couldn't possibly get any better, God showed me there was more. Each time one of my books is released, I watch as it moves up the Amazon bestsellers list. I read the e-mails from people who love my books and thank me for touching their lives. I revel in the fact that my God always has a plan and purpose for everything He does in my life. Everything happens in His time and according to His will. We cannot get ahead of Him, nor can we do it ourselves. I'm guilty of leaping when I should stand still and wait for His instructions.

Now and again, we look at situations and believe we have failed, but what we don't realize is that the process hasn't been completed yet. It took that e-mail for me to be able to put my writing career in God's hands—according to His will. No, the agent didn't sell my book or agree to represent me, but He did help me to humble my heart and realize that the only way to succeed is through God. He helped me to pray.

The day my books first arrived in the mail was one of the greatest days of my life. I held them in my hands and cried. Turning the pages, I just sobbed. As I looked at little Zippy and all of his beautiful pages, I experienced the blissful moment of happy tears.

Way back before Zippy was ever published, the first time I envisioned my little zebra without stripes, knowing I was the one who decided to make him different, broke my heart. Back then, I wanted to change the whole story and give him stripes. But then the Lord intervened and gave me another glimpse. In my heart I was able to see a zebra with the ability to help children. He was no longer lacking anything in my eyes. After seeing Zippy on the pages of my published book, I pulled out the box of rejection letters that had once been so hard for me to read, and I saw them with new understanding. I literally wanted to send every one of them a thank-you card and a big hug. If Zippy had been published years ago, like I'd wanted, he wouldn't have been as special. I know this because God blessed me to rewrite his story the night before I e-mailed it to ShadeTree.

God showed me we need to do everything possible for us to do and leave the impossible to Him. He writes the most beautiful stories with our lives and makes our reality even better than our dreams—despite our circumstances.

Despite Your Circumstances

Do you have a dream today? Is there a desire inside you to make a difference and help others? Make a list of your dreams and then develop a plan to achieve them. With God's help you can accomplish far more than you ever imagined. Dream big and tell your story!

1.

2.

3.

4.

5.

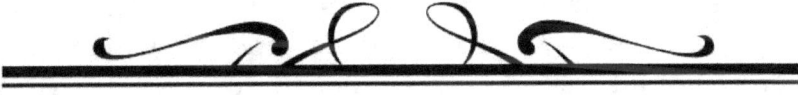

11
Fear

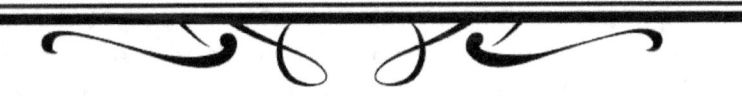

For God hath not given us the spirit of fear; but of power, and of love, and of a sound mind.
2 Timothy 1:7

Fear is a powerful emotion. It can overpower, paralyze, and even destroy us if we allow it to do so. The solution is to not give any type of terror or negative emotions control over our lives. The enemy works through our emotions.

Years ago, I was terrified of storms. I had some type of weather phobia, and if the forecast called for any type of bad weather, my whole week was ruined. I would pace the floors and tremble at the power of the storms. Then one day God showed me that He was in control.

Despite Your Circumstances

In the middle of a terrible storm, a tornado formed in our area. The wind outside was raging, and my anxiety was at an all-time high. Instead of easing, the wind intensified, and the sky began to growl as if it were outraged. I knew the funnel cloud was hovering over us, so I grabbed my children, knelt at the couch, and prayed.

The wind continued to howl, and hail battered the windows, but my fear was replaced with God's amazing peace. I was able to soothe my children because God had calmed me. The next day, as we surveyed the damage, we discovered several homes, barns, and trees that were destroyed all around us. Even though we were in the direct path of the tornado and in the very center of the storm, God spared us. Since that day, I haven't been afraid of the weather. Now I realize and know my God is in control of it all.

I have spent a great deal of time analyzing fear. I believe it comes from uncontrolled situations and is a spawn of the devil. It is a burden and a barrier to faith and the complete opposite of trust in God. When Peter had his eyes on Jesus, he was able to walk on the water. However, when the winds began to blow, he shifted his focus and became afraid. It was his fear that made him sink. As long as we keep our eyes on Jesus, we can do anything.

Recently, God has helped me overcome my dual phobias of public speaking and traveling. I remember the first time little Zippy and I ever visited a school. My body trembled and my mind conjured up horrible scenarios. Holding the book and turning the pages in front of people made me feel exposed and vulnerable. Having so many eyes on me at once was nerve-racking. And then there was the fear that no one would like my story.

In these times, we have to make a decision. We can either allow fear to dictate our lives and prevent us from following our dreams, or we can realize that courage is being scared and yet doing what we fear anyway. Once I decided to just do it, despite my fears, the most amazing thing happened. I looked over the crowd of smiling children, and my heart became thankful. It was so much fun sharing my story! Watching their expressions coincide with the story was amazing. Their sighs, expressions of sadness and joy, and laughter all touched my heart.

It is so precious to watch my story affect children—especially when I see their countenances change and I realize God is using me to help them. The gift of making a difference (big or small) in anyone's life is priceless and definitely trumps any fear.

Speaking at conferences was another matter entirely. Being the center of attention intimidated me and made me feel small. My self-worth was tested, along with my strength and my faith. I entertained thoughts like: *What in the world can I possibly share with college graduates and scholars they don't already know?* A multitude of questions raced through my thoughts and caused me tremendous stress.

A few days before my first conference, I developed a migraine. I had put so much pressure on myself to be perfect that my body rebelled. I prayed continuously and begged God to take away the pain. As my condition worsened, I wanted to withdraw myself from the event, but I knew that two hours of notice was not sufficient for them to find a replacement, so I had to go. The tears glided down my cheeks, reminding me of previous obstacles I had overcome. (My life is not always sunshine and gentle breezes. Sometimes it is downpours and thunderstorms, but that doesn't stop me from enjoying the rain.) I pleaded to God one last time, and then I picked up my cross, so to speak, and walked out my front door by faith. I was afraid, hurting, but most of all determined. I knew that if this trial derailed me, then the next one might destroy me.

When the coordinator introduced me to the audience, my vision blurred and my head pounded with each heartbeat. I couldn't see the words on my half-written speech. Feeling weak and vulnerable, I folded the paper and put it away. But then I opened my mouth and God's words tumbled out. He blessed me to testify of His greatness and all of the trials I had previously conquered. I stood in faith and trusted my God to see me through.

When the enemy attacked, God showed me that He is in control. He removed my thoughts and replaced them with His own. Serving God is not about winning or being better than anyone else. It is about doing His will. The crowd witnessed the misery etched on my face and knew I had persevered. My condition added power to the encouraging words. God blessed the event and even gave me additional opportunities. The next time, I conquered my fear with faith and realized that my opponent is powerless against God.

I also had to deal with my fear of traveling. My family and I had never been on a beach vacation before, but we had desired to go. Years prior, I blamed financial burdens for our lack of journeying. It was easier to blame expenses instead of admitting my fear of traveling. Occasionally, I would go on short trips, but my nerves still overwhelmed me. By the time we reached our destination, I would be a mess and the dread of driving home eclipsed any potential for fun.

When each of my books was released, I received several requests for out-of-town school visits. Reluctantly, I agreed. Coming home from one of them, the interstate had six lanes of traffic and I panicked. My sister was driving and my children were playing in the backseat. The fear tormented me, and I couldn't breathe. I wanted to stop, get out, and never travel again. Then I could hear my kids laughing. They were having fun and enjoying life with no worries. I wanted to be carefree, as well. In those moments, so many thoughts raced through my mind: *What are you so afraid of? Are you going to give the enemy the victory? Do you trust God? Do you really believe that He can take care of you?* My heart cried out, and God replaced my fear with peace. For the first time, I was surrounded by traffic and it had no control over me. I believed God would protect me and that even if we crashed, He would carry me home.

A few months later, we traveled to the beach without fear. We were driving through the mountains of North Carolina, trapped between a concrete wall and a tractor-trailer hauling a double-wide, and I just smiled. The perilous situation had no effect on me whatsoever. Even the enemy can't trouble God's stillness. Sometimes God puts us in situations where we have to step out of our comfort zones. In all reality, the safe havens we create for ourselves are not that helpful. They bind us and suppress our ability to grow and prosper accordingly. We all need to be pushed out of our safety zones every once in a while so that we can discover our true capabilities. I recently heard someone say, "The magic happens outside of our comfort zone."

Despite Your Circumstances

Through God we can be fearless. We need to take the first step by faith, knowing He will carry us the rest of the way. The only way the devil can defeat us is if we give up. God expects us to trust Him through each battle, obstacle, and trial life has to offer. Our flesh will always be consumed and tormented by some type of fear or heartache, but God's peace will soothe them all. I resolve to walk without fear—despite my circumstances.

Do you have any fears to conquer? Do you try to overcome your fears or do you allow them to defeat you? Make a list of your worries and challenges, and beside each one, add a promise from God that will help you to overcome it.

1.

2.

3.

4.

5.

12
Great Expectations

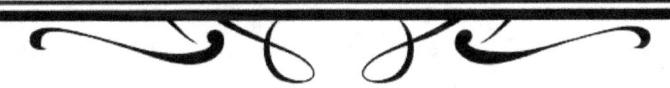

According to my earnest expectation and my hope, that in nothing I shall be ashamed, but that with all boldness, as always, so now also Christ shall be magnified in my body, whether it be by life, or by death.

Philippians 1:20

Most of the time I cause my own heartaches, especially when I expect too much of other people and assume they will act in a certain way. For example, I sometimes expect someone to do something special for me, but I become disappointed by their thoughtlessness when they don't comply with my preconceived wishes. What is even worse is when I've already done something special for them and then assume they will do the same for me. My biggest disappointment, however, takes place when I believe God should bless me in a certain way, but He doesn't.

We all expect more from people than they could ever give us. We build up great expectations for friends, family, and strangers. We even make up rules and think others should follow along. More often than not, we fail to give them a guide to our definition of "perfect," and then we change the guidelines as we go, neglecting to see the difficulty or impossibility that anyone could adhere to our specifications.

No one is perfect! And that's perfectly fine. It's when we expect them to be that a problem is created. Love should never be bound by strings and ultimatums. We should strive to love as our Father loves us. He knows our worth, and that our sins condemn us all. Still, He offers us the ultimate gift. The Lord bestowed on us the purest form of love, knowing we would still sin, turn away from Him and His love, disobey at every opportunity, and be ungrateful for His mercy and grace. Even so, God looks beyond our imperfections and sees something lovable in an unlovable form.

God looked at me and must have glimpsed someone weak and helpless—drowning in the midst of evil. My every move and thought was already known and understood by Him. God counted all the times I would fail and disappoint Him, but He chose to love me anyway. No strings! No conditions! No time frame! The purest affection ever created, and it goes on forever and ever, without pause. God showed us the perfect example of love, friendship, endurance, and forgiveness. Anything less is unacceptable. Unconditionally is how I try to love those in my life—as God has loved me.

When we're so busy expecting great things to happen, we often forget to be thankful for our present blessings. Here is a classic example: One year, because of recent sales and demands for my books, I placed a *huge* order of books to sell at a local festival. When I was determining what my order would be, I didn't know the weather was changing and it would be so hot that many people would stay home. God did know this, however, and He still urged me to order tons of books. As I sat at that festival and felt as if I were melting, all I could think about was the stack of unsold books. I was so focused on my own agenda that I failed to see God's blessings and purpose around me. Several days after the event, God showed me great blessings that I had originally missed. He reminded me of how when I read the story of Zippy, a change took place in a little girl listening and she found courage she didn't know existed. He also reminded me of how He had placed me beside the booth belonging to The Children's Reading Foundation of Appalachia. The leader and I bonded through the intense conditions and became friends. Soon after that, God blessed our paths to cross again and the foundation named me as their spokesperson for that year, thus opening so many beautiful opportunities to me. Even though I had great expectations to sell tons of books at the festival, God had even greater blessings for me. Through the foundation, different opportunities occurred over the course of the year, and I was able to connect with new people. Therefore, I ended up selling more books that I had originally planned. His ways are always greater and broader than we can even imagine. We should never allow our expectations to derail our journey.

Expectations go both ways, and we must learn to develop and lean on good ones. For example, I'm usually awakened by pain. Most days, it takes both therapy and ice to get me going. There are times when I have to wake up at 5 a.m. so that I can do all of the necessary stretches and tricks to be able to work that day. Nevertheless, every night when I go to sleep, I choose to expect that in the morning I will feel good despite what previous mornings have been like. I know that if I give up today, tomorrow it will be even easier to quit, and the next day it will require no effort at all to give up. Then I will be drowning in self-pity and become a burden to everyone around me. I don't want to be that kind of person. I have so much in my heart left to give. I enjoy living and working. So I fight, with everything inside me. I push until there's no strength left in my body, and then I push the hardest with my tears. I look to God during those painful moments and know that He will pick me up and carry me a little further.

I also know that God has expectations for me. He expects me to keep on keeping on. God wants me to keep getting up, regardless of how many times I get knocked down, and to continue even through the difficult periods. It pleases God for me to walk by faith and trust Him with my heartaches. He doesn't wish for me to accept defeat when life gets hard, but to continue trying even if it means crawling when I can't walk. Why? Because He knows the greatest testimony is given from the hearts of those who survived the storm, not merely those who heard about it.

We need to adopt higher expectations for ourselves and then be accountable for them. Excuses are stumbling blocks that over time will destroy us. If we cast the blame elsewhere for our wrongdoings, then we will never learn from our errors. Things don't occur because of luck; bad things usually happen because of wrong choices. When we learn to be the one always giving, then we are not as needy, because we change how we look at life and situations. If I focus all of my energy on being a good wife, then I don't concentrate my husband's shortcomings. If I am the kind of friend I want in return, there are no disappointments. When I strive to be a great mom, then my kids will blossom and grow.

I expect to do my best at all times. The quality of my work reflects the kind of person I am. Barely getting by doesn't satisfy my needs. We all need accomplishments to keep us motivated. If we can't find happiness in ourselves, then we shouldn't expect anyone or any relationship to give us what we are lacking. We can't expect to always get it right, though. Sometimes I try so hard, but I still fail. I don't like disappointing myself or God. It makes me feel horrible for my efforts to be void. If I don't reach my desired level of satisfaction, I tend to deem my labor as worthless, but I'm so thankful God sees things differently.

All God expects from us is obedience and trust. God understands my capabilities and needs better than anyone. If He allowed me to succeed with my every effort, I would become exalted in my works. My humbleness would be replaced with arrogance, and my reliance on Him would be forgotten. It is good for me to be sorrowful; that's when I pray and give others a little glimpse of my God. They see my struggles and then witness the power of God's assistance. Serving God and doing His work are not easy, but the rewards are amazing.

Instead of putting my trust and expectations in human beings, I try to put them in God. While I know God doesn't usually adhere to my guidelines, His capabilities greatly exceed any prospects or hope that I may have envisioned.

Despite Your Circumstances

God is the ultimate example of love, and because of Him I expect great things for my life—despite my circumstances.

Do you have any expectations and guidelines that need to be modified? Do people, God, and situations often disappoint you? Do you put restrictions on your love? Make a list of expectations you have that you want to change.

1.

2.

3.

4.

5.

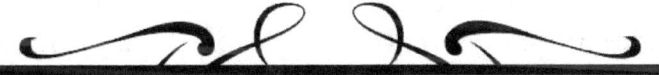

13
Suffering with a Smile

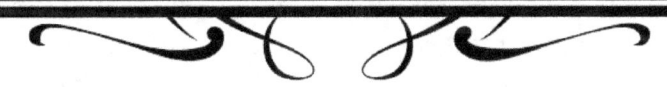

But and if ye suffer for righteousness' sake, happy are ye: and be not afraid of their terror, neither be troubled.

1 Peter 3:14

Life is one big lesson after another. It seems there are always obstacles to defeat and faith to exercise. My daddy said someone once told him, "It takes you a lifetime to learn how to live for the Lord, and by then, you're ready to go home." We may not always understand why, but God has a reason for each trial we experience. Our suffering is never in vain. God always rewards us for our heartaches. There is always a beautiful gift to be obtained.

Despite Your Circumstances

You can tell people all day long about God and His faithfulness, but sometimes you just need to show them. Allow them to see your smile despite the pain. Praise Him through the storms and give others a glimpse of His strength.

One day my sister and I were headed to lunch when my rib dislocated, leaving me with extreme pain and nausea. I wanted to curl up into a ball and cry. But since I knew crying about it wouldn't solve anything, I tried to smile and renew my positive thoughts. My sister looked at me and said, "How can you always smile and make light of what you go through?"

I thought about her question for a minute and swallowed my tears. "Sometimes I have to smile and laugh to keep from crying," I answered. If I cried every time I were in pain, I might never smile again. Wallowing in self-pity makes me sick of my own tears. Giving up every time hopelessness emerged would cause me to be one big crybaby. I'm not interested in that. I would rather smile.

I watch people's expressions and see when they notice the pain on my face. It hurts me even more to watch their smile fade as concern etches their features. Watching it affect my children is hard, too, especially when I cause them worry. I decided long ago that I will try to always smile and keep going—regardless of the situation.

When I was a little girl, the reactions of others broke my heart—it was unforgettable to see the horror on someone's face when they noticed my scars. Regardless of how many times it happened, it never became easier. One day, I asked God to give me something to distract them from my scars, something that would transform me from an ugly monster to a beautiful person in their eyes. And my Lord, being so understanding, gave me a smile.

Someone recently told me that when I smile, others get a glimpse of my soul. It has become my shield. Regardless of how badly I feel or how much my heart aches, I still smile—not just for me, but for others. When they think of me, I want them to remember that despite my circumstances and hardships, all is well with my soul.

When my days are challenging, I write in my gratitude journal. Making a list of my blessings puts my life in perspective, and helps me to realize that I have nothing to complain about. Gratitude triumphs over self-pity any day, and it always leaves me with a smile on my face.

Yes, I have pain, but I also have joy in my heart. It is up to me which one I concentrate on. If I focus on my pain and disabilities, then they multiply. On the contrary, if I focus on my abilities and my joy, then that will overcome my hardships.

One evening, when I was eating dinner, it became difficult for me to lift my hand to my mouth. The doctor said both of my shoulders were traumatized. Just the effort to feed myself made my eyes sting with tears. Knowing that I had a speaking event afterward made the tasks seem even more difficult. I wondered how I would be able to drive to and from the event and talk for an hour, all the while in severe pain. Then God changed everything.

God gave me a thought that changed my situation: I am a child of the King, I know God, and He loves me unconditionally. My God knows my name, and He has a plan for all of my hardships. He uses my challenges to help others. When I find joy and thankfulness during my suffering, the enemy is defeated. It pleases my heart that

God would even allow me to suffer for Him. It is my joy during the trials to reflect my God.

As His calming Spirit filled my soul, I was able to overcome my sorrows with joy. The best part, however, was the smile on my face and the connection I made with the audience. Someone even told me that when I spoke about my pain, my story touched his soul in an amazing way and showed him how to overcome his own trials. Once again God helped me to smile through my pain—despite my circumstances.

Do you embrace self-pity during difficult times, or do you look for the blessings among the trials? Make a list of ways you can learn to smile through your hardships.

1.

2.

3.

4.

5.

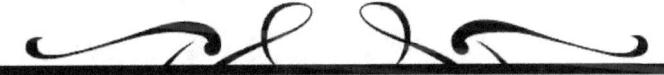

14
Unconditional Happiness

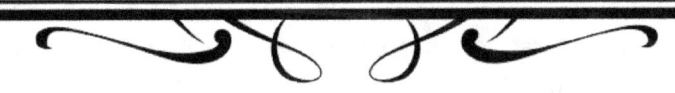

Happy is he that hath the God of Jacob for his help, whose hope is in the LORD his God.
Psalm 146:5

Have you ever thought, if only a certain something would happen, then you would be happy? I did. I constantly put limitations on my happiness and then wondered why I was so miserable. But I was the one who had decided not to be happy.

I remember thinking that if I could only get my books published, then I would be happy. After being published, though, I was bombarded with fear over the responsibilities of being an author. Another time I thought that if I didn't have a headache every day, I would be happy. But when my neck was finally better and my headaches stopped, my rib dislocated and caused me tremendous pain for almost a month. When my rib was finally healing, my hand decided to take a turn and start giving me grief. And then my legs started and I couldn't walk. I learned a very valuable lesson through it all: Be happy—despite the circumstances!

If we always wait for the stars to line up with the sun and the moon, for perfect weather, mood, body, and atmosphere in order to be happy, we will live a life of pure misery. Things will always go wrong and challenge us. However, that's what makes life interesting. If we keep our eyes on God, we won't faint when the hardships begin to surface. It's about training our minds to seek the bright side and hold on to the hope for a better day.

My sister and I were shopping once when it began to rain on our fun day. The rain was pouring from the sky. Other shoppers were standing inside the store complaining about the rain. But my sister and I took off running, and when we got to the car she started jumping in a puddle, as if that was the most normal thing in the world to do while it was raining. Everyone laughed. Sometimes we complain when we should be laughing.

We will always be challenged, have heartaches to overcome, find ourselves in situations that need modifications, and discover obstacles in our way. The key is going around, through, and over the top of them—with happiness. We shouldn't allow things to take away our ability to be happy. It's a choice. Don't be the negative person who brings everyone else down. Be the happy person whom everyone wants to be around. Sure, we all have bad days. We all experience sadness and feel defeated at times. It's okay to cry and pray, but self-pity is not allowed.

Circumstances do not need to define, break, or destroy us. They can strengthen and get us ready for the next battle. God doesn't punish us with hard times; He blesses us with them. It pleases Him to hear our voice of thankfulness during our trials. I believe it angers God to hear us complain relentlessly about our blessings, when we are never satisfied or content.

Complaining is nothing more than a bad habit. It is possible to train our minds to seek the positive thoughts and disregard the negative ones immediately. One day I met a woman who inspired me to never complain again. The moment she opened her mouth, a long list of negative, gloomy thoughts emerged. She frowned continuously and tried to make me see only the ugly side of life. It was enlightening to hear her complain insistently. With every criticism uttered, she ended with a question for me. I never opened my mouth and instead smiled at her the whole time. Actually, I was amazed that anyone could be so ungrateful. I didn't know how to respond, and I wasn't about to agree with her tirade. When she left, I vowed to never complain aloud to anyone again. Then the thought occurred to me: If one woman could choose to only see the bad in life, perhaps another could choose to only see the good. I wanted to be the happy woman without complaints—despite my circumstances.

Despite Your Circumstances

Do you choose happiness for your life? What are some ways in which you reaffirm your happiness daily?

1.

2.

3.

4.

5.

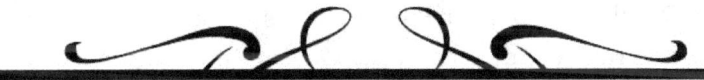

15
Bad Days

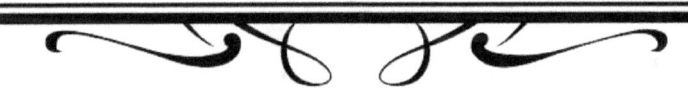

But the salvation of the righteous is of the LORD; he is their strength in the time of trouble.
Psalm 37:39

Sometimes we need to remember what is waiting on us. We need to glimpse, through an eye of faith, our hope of a better day. We can turn our bad days into good days—despite our circumstances.

Even when I feel bad, if I make an effort to be happy it helps me to overcome the heartache. On my desk, I have a list of positive actions to help me survive the bad days:

   ** Realize this heartache will soon pass. These feelings will not last forever.

Despite Your Circumstances

- ** Pray! First for me, and then for someone else.
- ** Remind myself that all things work together for my own good, and that God always knows what is best for me.
- ** Remember that the only way to truly pray is with a broken heart.
- ** Remember that the devil fights me the hardest when I'm doing something good for my Lord.
- ** Realize that we are given tests to see how we handle certain situations.
- ** Exercise. Sometimes a walk can do wonders for my body, which is hurting, and my mind, which is overwhelmed.
- ** Cry.
- ** Count my blessings.
- ** Read His beautiful words of power.
- ** Remember that God is always in control.
- ** Smile, whether I feel like it or not. A smile can be contagious and maybe someone else needs it, too.

What are some ways in which you conquer your bad days?

1.

2.

3.

4.

5.

Despite Your Circumstances

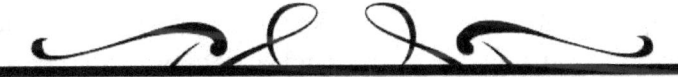

16
My Big Change

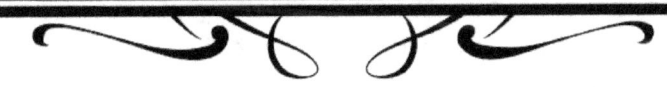

And we know that all things work together for the good to them that love God, to them who are the called according to his purpose.
                                    Romans 8:28

Just an FYI: If you don't want people to stare at you or your scars, then you shouldn't write a book about them and appear in newspapers and television interviews! I learned this the hard way.

When my books first came out, my life changed dramatically. All of a sudden, *everyone* was looking at me. People stopped in the aisles of stores and openly stared at me. It made me want to crawl back into my shell. I wanted to shove my hands in my pockets all over again and hide. But I soon realized that I had come too far to quit.

So I smiled and answered their questions. Most people had never noticed me before. I didn't even flinch (well, I hope not, anyway!) when I was called "handicapped" and "disabled," "disfigured," and "deformed." I realized that sometimes we have to go through the bad to get to the good.

In order to share my story and help others, I had to go through every step of the process. I had to talk about my heartaches and fears, and somehow become a voice as well as an image for those who are different. God has given me an amazing opportunity. Most people just simply do not know about certain syndromes or challenges. All they know is what they have assumed or been told. I feel it is important for me to tell others about amniotic band syndrome and how it has personally affected me. God always provides me with the perfect words to explain what people need to hear.

All anyone needs is the right perspective. For example, one day I saw a child who was covered in bandages and being pushed in a wheelchair. My first response was such pity and heartache that I cried. But as I walked to my car, grieving for this child, God stopped me. He reminded me that the child was alive—to love and be loved. Physical scars do not change the feelings of the heart. It doesn't affect the ability to love at all. Scars mean we survived the trauma. They mean God blessed us with mercy and love. They are a reminder of what we suffered and how we prevailed.

It's the way we choose to look at a situation that defines it. We can look at someone who is wounded and scarred and pity them, or we can look at them and know that God is merciful and loving. I think things sometimes happen to get our attention. Events happen without explanations or plausible cause in order to give us a glimpse of the grandeur of God's ways.

It is impossible to believe in miracles without ever hearing about or seeing them. They become our sunbeams during dark, cloudy days. We all need something to make us believe in the unbelievable. Troubles make us stop, examine our lives, and count our blessings. Tragedy changes how we view our lives. Heartbreak helps us to sort our lives with a greater sense of importance.

If perfection is our view of a great life, then it's obscured and hopeless. We need to remember all the different colors needed to make a beautiful rainbow. Different shapes and sizes make the most beautiful flower garden. All different kinds of people make the world lovely. If we were all the same, there would be no array of beautiful. There would be no glimpses of miracles, the extraordinary, the amazing, or even God. We need diversity to make us stop every once in a while and evaluate our views on life. We need those moments to surprise us and make us believe in things greater than the eye can see. We need to be reminded of God's mercy and the grace that surrounds us all.

Different is not ugly, shameful, or hopeless. Different is beautiful! It is miraculous, wonderful, incredible, wondrous, extraordinary, and phenomenal. We are all amazing—the way God created each and every one of us. We should never dwell on our flaws, but rather celebrate our differences.

What we may criticize as a mistake, may be a blessing. I have always disliked the scar on my right arm. The amniotic band wrapped around it and caused a visual impression. People stop me in stores and instruct me to remove the band before it cuts my arm off. When I tell them it's a scar, it makes us both feel uncomfortable for a moment. Then one day, I looked at my scar with a new perspective. The band could have amputated my arm near the shoulder. Instead it only left a mark of its presence. Now when I look at my arm, I'm so thankful God blessed me to keep it to hold the scar.

With total acceptance I'm able to praise my Lord. I no longer whine about what was taken away or scarred, but I'm thankful for everything God blessed me to keep. I am changed—despite my circumstances.

Is there a situation in your life that needs a new perspective? Make a list of any thoughts, feelings, or circumstances that burden your life. Now create a new outlook on those burdens.

1.

2.

3.

4.

5.

Candida Sullivan

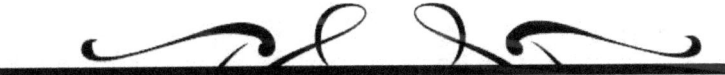

Favorite Scriptures

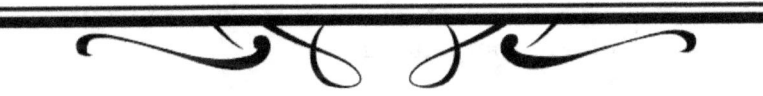

We all go through hard times and struggle to keep moving forward. When heartaches emerge in my life, the need for comfort becomes automatic and I start searching the scriptures. I desire wholeheartedly for God to reassure me that my problem won't defeat me. His words of encouragement and love soothe my troubled soul.

I have compiled a list of my favorite verses that have helped me through so many difficult times. I pray these scriptures will help you as much as they have helped me.

Adversity

1 Peter 1:7
That the trial of your faith, being much more precious than of gold that perisheth, though it be tried with fire, might be found unto praise and honour and glory at the appearing of Jesus Christ.

John 16:33
These things I have spoken unto you, that in me ye might have peace. In the world ye shall have tribulation: but be of good cheer; I have overcome the world.

Romans 8:18
For I reckon that the sufferings of this present time are not worthy to be compared with the glory which shall be revealed in us.

Nahum 1:7
The LORD is good, a strong hold in the day of trouble; and he knoweth them that trust in him.

Anger

Romans 12:19-21
Dearly beloved, avenge not yourselves, but rather give place unto wrath: for it is written, Vengeance is mine; I will repay, saith the Lord. Therefore if thine enemy hunger, feed him; if he thirst, give him drink: for in so doing thou shalt heap coals of fire on his head. Be not overcome of evil, but overcome evil with good.

Ephesians 4:26
Be ye angry, and sin not: let not the sun go down upon your wrath.

Ephesians 4:31-32
Let all bitterness, and wrath, and anger, and clamour, and evil speaking, be put away from you, with all malice: And be ye kind one to another, tenderhearted, forgiving one another, even as God for Christ's sake hath forgiven you.

Proverbs 16:32
He that is slow to anger is better than the mighty; and he that ruleth his spirit than he that taketh a city.

Comfort

Isaiah 40:31
But they that wait upon the LORD shall renew their strength; they shall mount up with wings as eagles; they shall run, and not be weary; and they shall walk, and not faint.

Matthew 5:4
Blessed are they that mourn: for they shall be comforted.

Psalm 23:4
Yea, though I walk through the valley of the shadow of death, I will fear no evil: for thou art with me; thy rod and thy staff they comfort me.

Psalm 30:5
For his anger endureth but a moment; in his favour is life: weeping may endure for a night, but joy cometh in the morning.

Courage

Isaiah 40:29
He giveth power to the faint; and to them that have no might he increaseth strength.

Psalm 31:24
Be of good courage, and he shall strengthen your heart, all ye that hope in the LORD.

Hebrews 13:6
So that we may boldly say, The Lord is my helper, and I will not fear what man shall do unto me.

Ephesians 3:12
In whom we have boldness and access with confidence by the faith of him.

Encouragement

Philippians 4:13
I can do all things through Christ which strengtheneth me.

Luke 22:32
But I have prayed for thee, that thy faith fail not: and when thou art converted, strengthen thy brethren.

James 4:7
Submit yourselves therefore to God. Resist the devil, and he will flee from you.

Luke 18:27
And he said, The things which are impossible with men are possible with God.

Faith

1 Corinthians 2:5
That your faith should not stand in the wisdom of men, but in the power of God.

Galatians 3:26
For ye are all the children of God by faith in Christ Jesus.

Mark 9:23
Jesus said unto him, If thou canst believe, all things are possible to him that believeth.

Mark 11:22-23
And Jesus answering saith unto them, Have faith in God. For verily I say unto you, That whosoever shall say unto this mountain, Be thou removed, and be thou cast into the sea; and shall not doubt in his heart, but shall believe that

those things which he saith shall come to pass; he shall have whatsoever he saith.

Fear

Isaiah 43:2
When thou passest through the waters, I will be with thee; and through the rivers, they shall not overflow thee: when thou walkest through the fire, thou shalt not be burned; neither shall the flame kindle upon thee.

1 Peter 3:12–14
For the eyes of the Lord are over the righteous, and his ears are open unto their prayers: but the face of the Lord is against them that do evil. And who is he that will harm you, if ye be followers of that which is good? But and if ye suffer for righteousness' sake, happy are ye: and be not afraid of their terror, neither be troubled.

Matthew 10:28
And fear not them which kill the body, but are not able to kill the soul: but rather fear him which is able to destroy both soul and body in hell.

John 14:27
Peace I leave with you, my peace I give unto you: not as the world giveth, give I unto you. Let not your heart be troubled, neither let it be afraid.

Guidance

Proverbs 3:6
In all thy ways acknowledge him, and he shall direct thy paths.

Psalm 37:23
The steps of a good man are ordered by the LORD: and he delighteth in his way.

Despite Your Circumstances

Isaiah 30:21
And thine ears shall hear a word behind thee, saying, This is the way, walk ye in it, when ye turn to the right hand, and when ye turn to the left.

John 16:13
Howbeit when he, the Spirit of truth, is come, he will guide you into all truth: for he shall not speak of himself; but whatsoever he shall hear, that shall he speak: and he will shew you things to come.

Hope

Jeremiah 17:7
Blessed is the man that trusteth in the LORD, and whose hope the LORD is.

Philippians 1:20
According to my earnest expectation and my hope, that in nothing I shall be ashamed, but that with all boldness, as always, so now also Christ shall be magnified in my body, whether it be by life, or by death.

Galatians 5:5
For we through the Spirit wait for the hope of righteousness by faith.

Psalm 71:5
For thou art my hope, O Lord GOD: thou art my trust from my youth.

Humility

James 4:10
Humble yourselves in the sight of the Lord, and he shall lift you up.

Proverbs 15:33
The fear of the LORD is the instruction of wisdom; and before honour is humility.

Matthew 23:12
And whosoever shall exalt himself shall be abased; and he that shall humble himself shall be exalted.

Proverbs 27:2
Let another man praise thee, and not thine own mouth; a stranger, and not thine own lips.

Love of God

John 3:16
For God so loved the world, that he gave his only begotten Son, that whosoever believeth in him should not perish, but have everlasting life.

1 Corinthians 13:13
And now abideth faith, hope, charity, these three; but the greatest of these is charity.

1 Thessalonians 4:9
But as touching brotherly love ye need not that I write unto you: for ye yourselves are taught of God to love one another.

Romans 12:10
Be kindly affectioned one to another with brotherly love; in honour preferring one another.

Mercy

Job 11:6
And that he would shew thee the secrets of wisdom, that they are double to that which is! Know therefore that God exacteth of thee less than thine iniquity deserveth.

Psalm 86:15
But thou, O Lord, art a God full of compassion, and gracious, longsuffering, and plenteous in mercy and truth.

Exodus 33:19
And he said, I will make all my goodness pass before thee, and I will proclaim the name of the LORD before thee; and will be gracious to whom I will be gracious, and will shew mercy on whom I will shew mercy.

Luke 6:36
Be ye therefore merciful, as your Father also is merciful.

Obedience

Deuteronomy 29:9
Keep therefore the words of this covenant, and do them, that ye may prosper in all that ye do.

Job 36:11
If they obey and serve him, they shall spend their days in prosperity, and their years in pleasures.

Proverbs 3:1–4
My son, forget not my law; but let thine heart keep my commandments: For length of days, and long life, and peace, shall they add to thee. Let not mercy and truth forsake thee: bind them about thy neck; write them upon the table of thine heart: So shalt thou find favour and good understanding in the sight of God and man.

1 Samuel 15:22
And Samuel said, Hath the LORD as great delight in burnt offerings and sacrifices, as in obeying the voice of the LORD? Behold, to obey is better than sacrifice, and to hearken than the fat of rams.

Patience

Galatians 6:9
And let us not be weary in well doing: for in due season we shall reap, if we faint not.

James 1:3-4
Knowing this, that the trying of your faith worketh patience. But let patience have her perfect work, that ye may be perfect and entire, wanting nothing.

Hebrews 12:1
Wherefore seeing we also are compassed about with so great a cloud of witnesses, let us lay aside every weight, and the sin which doth so easily beset us, and let us run with patience the race that is set before us,

Romans 5:3-5
And not only so, but we glory in tribulations also: knowing that tribulation worketh patience; And patience, experience; and experience, hope: And hope maketh not ashamed; because the love of God is shed abroad in our hearts by the Holy Ghost which is given unto us.

Perseverance

Romans 8:35
Who shall separate us from the love of Christ? shall tribulation, or distress, or persecution, or famine, or nakedness, or peril, or sword?

Revelation 3:21
To him that overcometh will I grant to sit with me in my throne, even as I also overcame, and am set down with my Father in his throne.

Ephesians 6:13
Wherefore take unto you the whole armour of God, that ye may be able to withstand in the evil day, and having done all, to stand.

Hebrews 10:23
Let us hold fast the profession of our faith without wavering; (for he is faithful that promised).

Prayer

Romans 8:26
Likewise the Spirit also helpeth our infirmities: for we know not what we should pray for as we ought: but the Spirit itself maketh intercession for us with groanings which cannot be uttered.

Jeremiah 29:12
Then shall ye call upon me, and ye shall go and pray unto me, and I will hearken unto you.

Isaiah 65:24
And it shall come to pass, that before they call, I will answer; and while they are yet speaking, I will hear.

1 John 5:14–15
And this is the confidence that we have in him, that, if we ask any thing according to his will, he heareth us: And if we know that he hear us, whatsoever we ask, we know that we have the petitions that we desired of him.

Strength

Psalm 18:2
The LORD is my rock, and my fortress, and my deliverer; my God, my strength, in whom I will trust; my buckler, and the horn of my salvation, and my high tower.

2 Corinthians 12:9
And he said unto me, My grace is sufficient for thee: for my strength is made perfect in weakness. Most gladly therefore will I rather glory in my infirmities, that the power of Christ may rest upon me.

Ephesians 6:10
Finally, my brethren, be strong in the Lord, and in the power of his might.

Colossians 1:10–11
That ye might walk worthy of the Lord unto all pleasing, being fruitful in every good work, and increasing in the knowledge of God; Strengthened with all might, according to his glorious power, unto all patience and longsuffering with joyfulness.

Success

Psalm 128:2
For thou shalt eat the labour of thine hands: happy shalt thou be, and it shall be well with thee.

Deuteronomy 16:15
Seven days shalt thou keep a solemn feast unto the LORD thy God in the place which the LORD shall choose: because the LORD thy God shall bless thee in all thine increase, and in all the works of thine hands, therefore thou shalt surely rejoice.

2 Chronicles 15:7
Be ye strong therefore, and let not your hands be weak: for your work shall be rewarded.

Colossians 1:10
That ye might walk worthy of the Lord unto all pleasing, being fruitful in every good work, and increasing in the knowledge of God.

Trust

Psalm 37:4–5
Delight thyself also in the LORD; and he shall give thee the desires of thine heart. Commit thy way unto the LORD; trust also in him; and he shall bring it to pass.

Despite Your Circumstances

Proverbs 3:5–6
Trust in the LORD with all thine heart; and lean not unto thine own understanding. In all thy ways acknowledge him, and he shall direct thy paths.

Isaiah 46:4
And even to your old age I am he; and even to hoar hairs will I carry you: I have made, and I will bear; even I will carry, and will deliver you.

Romans 8:28
And we know that all things work together for good to them that love God, to them who are the called according to his purpose.

About the Author

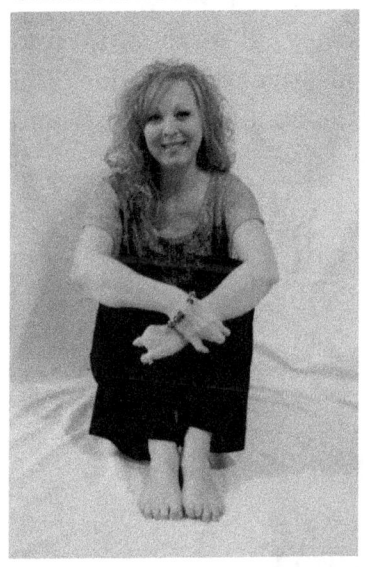

CANDIDA SULLIVAN believes in miracles. She was born with a rare condition called amniotic band syndrome, which generally causes death in most babies before they are ever born. She knows that it is a beautiful blessing that she survived, and she wants to show the world that her scars are not a punishment, but instead are a wonderful expression of God's love and mercy for her life. She believes God spared her for a reason, and she wants to spend her life telling of the hope and love God placed inside of her.

Candida also believes in dreams. Her first two books, *Zippy and the Stripes of Courage* and *Underneath the Scars*, were finalists in the 2012 Readers Favorite Award and nominated for the 2013 Christian Small Publishers Association Book of the Year Award. Candida was also chosen as the spokesperson for the Children's Reading Foundation of Appalachia, Kentucky, for 2013. She knows God makes the reality even better than the dreams.

Candida lives in Tennessee with her husband, Shannon, and her two boys, Cayden and Jordon. She teaches Sunday school and loves to be surrounded by the wonder and excitement of kids.

See Zippy in his first book titled *Zippy and the Stripes of Courage,* his second one titled *Zippy's Big Difference*, and his third one titled *Zippy's Club.* See also Candida's book for adults, *Underneath the Scars*, for her story of overcoming the effects of amniotic band syndrome.

Despite Your Circumstances

Other Books by Candida

Underneath the Scars is a journey of emotional and spiritual healing associated with physical deformities. You will laugh, cry, and reflect as Candida shares her story and the woman underneath her scars.

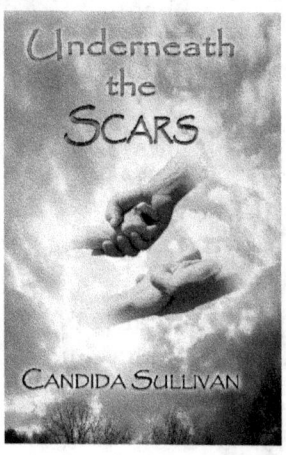

Candida Sullivan

Zippy and the Stripes of Courage is a story about how Zippy the zebra came to accept himself for who he is. It teaches children to celebrate one another's differences and to treat others as they themselves want to be treated.

English　　　　Spanish

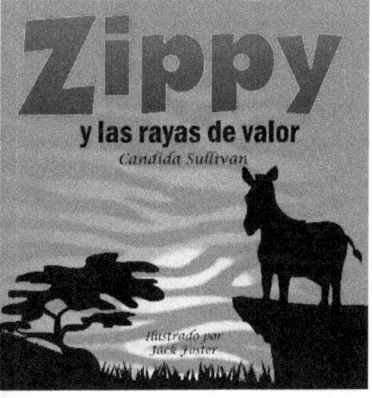

Zippy's Big Difference is a story about how Zippy the zebra came to appreciate that which makes him different from others. It deals with the emotional struggles facing children with disabilities and tackles some of the tough spiritual questions they have.

English   Spanish

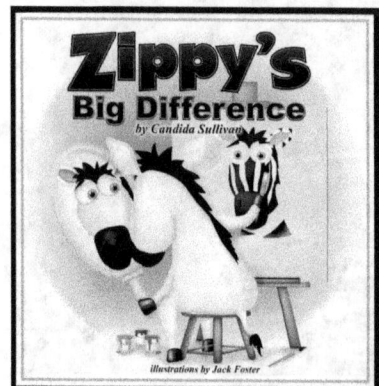 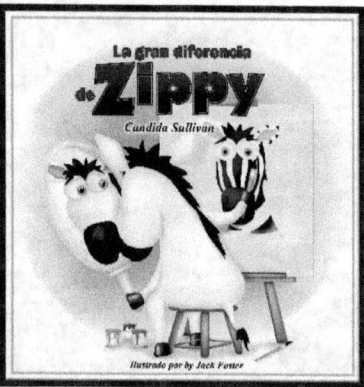

Zippy's Club invites kids to be part of the anti-bullying team. It teaches them to overcome bullying with kindness and to celebrate one another's differences. The book includes a section from a nationally certified counselor to help initiate conversations with kids about bullying, as well as a letter from Candida telling her personal story.

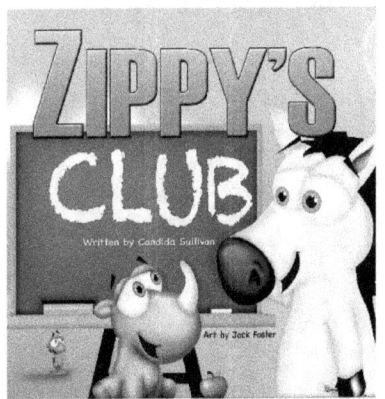

The *Zippy Club Kit* is a resource to go along with the books and can be used in classrooms to promote the anti-bullying message. The kit includes the following:

- ** A printed and digital full script of *Zippy's Club (The Play)*, which can be performed in classrooms
- ** A CD of masks for all the Zippy book characters
- ** Printable coloring sheets and stickers
- ** A Zippy Club poster, badge, and membership certificate

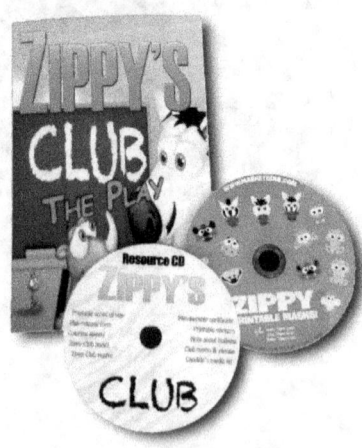

Candida Sullivan

About Amniotic Band Syndrome

Amniotic band syndrome (ABS) is a rare condition caused by string-like bands in the amniotic sac. These bands can entangle the umbilical cord or other parts of the baby's body. The constriction can cause a variety of problems depending on where they are located and how tightly they are wrapped. The complications from ABS vary. Mild banding can result in amputation or scarring, while severe banding can result in the death of the baby.

The medical community cannot truly explain what causes amniotic bands to form. While some call it a fluke of nature, I believe it is a symbol of God's amazing, miraculous love. God doesn't punish us with scars; He blesses us with life. The scars show the world that there is a God and that He is great.

Author's Acknowledgments

I would like to thank God, foremost—the center of my life. My God exemplifies everything wonderful, beautiful, great, and loving in my life. He has blessed me so greatly. Thank You, God, for allowing me to write more books and for all of the hearts they have touched. Thank You for allowing me to visit schools and for all of the ones we have helped. Thank You for showing me how to be an overcomer and how to be happy despite my circumstances. Most of all, thank You for loving me and allowing me to live. Thank You, God, for giving me scars to remind me of Your great love and mercy for me and my life.

Thank you to everyone who has read my books and offered your wonderful support. Thank you to all of the schools, classrooms, and homes who have welcomed us so greatly; who read my books over and over to their children; who shared their stories of struggle and triumph with me; who supported my books and made them so successful. Thank you for your prayers, kindness, love, and support. You will never know how much you mean to me.

Thank you to ShadeTree Publishing for making every part of this journey so wonderful! Thank you for caring about me as well as my cause and for working so hard to make it all happen. Thank you for always pushing me to do my best, and for making me dig deeper to find the real story.

Last but not least, thank you to my family. I couldn't do any of this without you! It's because of your love, prayers, and all of the special things you do to help me that I'm able to live my dreams.